The Kegel Legacy

The Kegel Legacy

Barry Fowler

First published in the UK by The Cloister House Press

ISBN 978-1-909465-13-8

Contents

Thanks to Sue, Rebecca, Anne and Janey
for your support and help

Foreword

I never guessed that a chance meeting in 1997 with Susie Hewson, the inspirational entrepreneur and founder of Natracare™, would change my whole career path and indeed my whole life. Meeting her, I realised that an individual with passion and strong beliefs, and a clear focus, can make a difference. It soon became clear to me that someone needed to make a difference in the way that incontinence was being treated and, in the absence of any other champion, I seem to have taken on that role.

Within a week or two of first meeting Susie I had set up a new company to promote the use of her natural, organic and biodegradable sanitary products. I was soon campaigning to bring a range of healthier and more environmentally-sound products to a wider audience.

As I carried out research to broaden my knowledge of these new markets it became very apparent that something was amiss. Why were over 20% of sanitary pad sales being used by women to manage the symptoms of their stress incontinence? And more especially, why were there so many millions of women with the problem anyway, when a highly effective cure was fully documented in the medical literature.

The answer seems clear to me – the taboo nature of Urinary Stress Incontinence means it is a subject not easily raised by the sufferers themselves or by those best placed to help them. Though well-meaning, the exercises recommended by doctors and physiotherapists as the first line of treatment, and information in the media, bear little resemblance to the pioneering work done by Arnold Kegel – even though modern pelvic floor exercises bear his name.

Most critically, the recommended 'modern' treatment is clearly inadequate, not fit for purpose, and leaves most women no better off, feeling frustrated and helpless.

So I began a personal mission to promote a more effective form of exercise, based on Kegel's clearly effective principles. My goal is that women will realise that they do not need to suffer from health problems such as incontinence and prolapse and that they can do so much, with the appropriate information, to help themselves.

It has not been a quick or simple task. In the process I have developed an exercise device which, at the time of writing, remains the only clinically proven pelvic toning device available on GP prescription in the UK.

Nothing is quick or simple. Despite extraordinary enthusiasm from the Professors of Urology when they first saw the PelvicToner™, it took nearly four years to set up and complete the UK clinical trial and a further year to get the device onto the UK Drug Tariff – the list of prescription products.

The job is far from complete. Far too many people in the medical profession, the media and the general public are still unaware of, or blind to, the health consequences of childbirth and the menopause and the effective treatments that are available. To say that there is a wall of indifference is an understatement. This book is just the latest of many steps to improve that awareness.

I am indebted to the thousands of women over the years who have taken the time to talk to me and explain their hopes, fears and frustrations and to share their joy at finding a cure. This book is dedicated to them.

Barry Fowler
May 2013

Chapter 1
Introduction

Incontinence is a significant worldwide problem

- Over 200 million women worldwide suffer from incontinence
- It is estimated that between 5 and 7 million women in the UK suffered incontinence in the past year
- Embarrassing leaks due to Stress incontinence affect one in three to a half of all new mothers
- The underlying cause, pelvic floor weakness, is easily rectified
- The help and advice being offered to women is clearly failing to address the problem

The lost cure

65 years ago a renowned doctor put his name to a proven treatment for a range of health problems that affect the majority of women after childbirth:

- the embarrassment of incontinence
- the discomfort and pain of prolapse
- the frustration of an impaired sex life

For 65 years women have been denied accurate and meaningful information about this treatment by the people they should trust – doctors and the media.

Today we have the most sophisticated and inclusive media of all time but most women are still unaware of the facts. As a result, millions suffer on a daily basis.

1

And at the same time a multibillion industry has grown to feed on the largely unnecessary, and the newly acquired, 'need' for designer incontinence pads.

How can this have possibly come about and why is no-one interested?

Oh! The memories

Most women have heard the word 'Kegel' in the context of pelvic floor exercises and it may have positive or negative connotations for them. It may bring back memories of the joyous birth of a baby and the start of a new family. Or it may be a reminder to do the pelvic floor squeezes that the midwife mentioned which you never really have time for and, besides, they never seemed to do much anyway.

What most women will not appreciate is that the pelvic floor exercises that bear the name 'Kegel' were first proposed by a doctor called Arnold Kegel who spent his lifetime trying to cure women of health conditions that, even today, cause embarrassment and discomfort to hundreds of millions of women around the world.

And the reason why so many women still suffer these totally curable problems is simple. For reasons this book explores, the exercises developed by Arnold Kegel, and tested on thousands of women over many decades, were totally ignored by the medical profession and the media for many years until they were replaced by a pale imitation of the rigorous and effective system that was intended.

You couldn't make it up

Or could you? Let us try and place the Kegel story in a more modern context. Imagine the scene:

An enthusiastic researcher presents his ideas to the panel of medical experts and investors on the reality TV show "This Doctor's Got Talent".

He has been working for 18 years to understand why so

2

many women suffer so many problems following the natural process of childbirth.

Following clinical trials with thousands of patients he has developed a cheap easy-to-use solution - a simple exercise device that delivers excellent results when used for an hour every day.

The panel are really impressed but point out that there just isn't the money to give every patient their own device. So they decide to drop that idea.

The therapists who will actually dispense the treatment are convinced that they do not need a machine anyway They do not believe that anyone would spend an hour a day doing exercises, so they reduce the time to just five minutes.

The PR specialists and the spin doctors see all this as a real challenge. How do you get the message across to all the affected individuals when urine leaks are such an embarrassing thing to talk about?

Meanwhile, in the absence of an effective treatment, the manufacturers of incontinence pads look forward to the prospect of an ever increasing market and spending their multimillion advertising budgets.

Before and after

In essence this is could be uncomfortably close to the truth!

Based on decades of research and trials with thousands of women, Arnold Kegel recommended an exercise regime that comprised 20 minutes of exercise three times a day and each session of exercise involved about 300 squeezes against the maximum resistance the patient could manage using a special resistance measuring device.

By comparison, the exercise routines currently recommended by the National Institute for Health and Clinical Excellence (NICE) who set the standards for treatment in the UK are for *"8 contractions three times a day. Continue for three months"*. The UK Chartered

Society of Physiotherapy says *"Squeeze and lift as strongly as you can. Hold for ten seconds. Relax for ten seconds. Repeat ten times. Follow with ten fast squeezes as fast as you can".* There is no mention of squeezing anything other than thin air.

Kegel observed objective or measurable improvement in two weeks with "good urinary control in 84% of patients". This is still held up as the yardstick for what pelvic floor exercise can achieve. However, in 2013 it is estimated that up to half of women who have had children will suffer incontinence, if not in the years following childbirth then after menopause. The two statistics must be linked to the comparative effectiveness of the two exercise regimes.

To put these figures into sharp focus, clinical research indicates that at least a third of new mothers will suffer from stress incontinence. This represents 5,000 women every week adding to a population of between 5 and 7 million sufferers across the UK.

When, where and how did the rigour of Kegel's proposals get so watered down? And why?

The forgotten muscle

To understand the importance of Kegel exercises it is necessary to understand a little about your anatomy.

The pelvic floor or pelvic diaphragm is responsible for holding all the pelvic organs within the bony structures of the pelvis. The pelvic floor supports the weight of all your internal organs. It is through your pelvic floor that your anus, vagina and urethra meet the outside world.

You will be vaguely aware of your pelvic floor and you can feel where it is and what it is doing in two ways. Firstly, when you need to pass urine, sit on the toilet with your legs apart and see if you can start and then stop the flow of urine without moving your legs. If you can stop the stream of urine, you are tightening the main pelvic floor muscle. If you can restart the stream of urine, you are relaxing the correct muscle.

It is the same muscle that you would use if you wanted to avoid breaking wind in public!

Secondly, you can insert a finger into your vagina, and try to tighten the muscles around your finger as if holding back urine. You should feel a pressure or squeeze along the length of your finger.

Clinical studies show that about a third of women cannot identify and squeeze their pelvic floor. There are a number of reasons for this but the main one is that the pelvic floor is 'out of sight, out of mind'. The fact is that for most women it is underused and under-exercised and, as a result, the muscle has never 'learnt' to squeeze on demand and the link between the brain and the muscle is not sufficiently developed.

Poor sex and embarrassing health problems

When the pelvic floor muscle weakens, atrophies or is damaged, for example in childbirth, a number of things can happen. If the vaginal muscle becomes weak and flaccid there is a decrease in sexual pleasure for both partners caused, in part, by a lack of good intimate contact during intercourse.

More seriously, you may develop urinary or stool incontinence, that is, an inability to control the bladder or bowel. And without the appropriate muscular support there can be a prolapse which is a falling down or slipping out of place of the internal organs. This is an uncomfortable condition in which the bladder, rectum, or uterus move down into the vagina or begin to bulge through the walls of the vagina. We will discuss this more later.

There are two life stage events that specifically affect the pelvic floor: childbirth and the menopause. However, obesity and a general lack of fitness are also significant factors when it comes to health issues caused by pelvic floor weakness.

Arnold Kegel proved that a series of very simple exercises could firstly restore muscle tone in cases where this muscle was weakened and atrophied, and could also significantly strengthen the weakened muscle.

Over the coming pages we will explore what Arnold Kegel actually recommended and why. In particular we will look at the health improvements he achieved in women of all ages. And then explore why doctors, physiotherapists, midwives and health writers appear to have failed to make women aware of the simple, effective technique that could cure their problems.

My aim in writing this book is to empower women by providing information about past research and current products that are now available, including one I have personally developed (more of that later. See Chapter 9). Armed with this knowledge, women who may need help will be better informed of the best way forward.

Kegel and his exercises

Arnold Kegel first introduced a simple, effective clinically proven treatment for weak pelvic floor muscles in 1948 but his work was largely ignored. The first recorded use of the phrase 'Kegel Exercises' is in 1975 (Merriam-Webster online dictionary), nearly 30 years after his principles were first documented in the medical literature.

The basic principles identified by Arnold Kegel were fundamental to the success he achieved but the exercises that now bear his name, as promoted by health professionals and the media, bear no relationship to the rigorous techniques he originally identified. As a result, millions of women suffer the long term consequences.

Arnold Kegel offered enormous hope to millions of women and he should be ranked amongst the greats of medicine and science. Instead his legacy is in danger of being totally ignored.

If you were a conspiracy theorist you could be forgiven for thinking that Kegel was the subject of a conspiracy of silence. But there is only an element of conspiracy. The greater factor is that his proposals were just forgotten for 30 years and when the idea of exercise became topical again everyone came up with new ideas and no-one went back and tested them against the best benchmark they had.

How have we reached this situation? And what can women do to take control of the situation and overcome one of the last remaining taboos of the 21st Century? That is the objective of this book.

65 years of denial

Why denial? 65 years after Arnold Kegel first announced the results of his extensive research:

• Women are still in denial about, or ignorant of, the long term health problems of natural childbirth including urinary incontinence, prolapse and sexual dysfunction
• The medical professionals involved are in denial and have persisted with a treatment that is not solving the problems caused by pelvic floor weakness and is clearly not fit for purpose. There has been no systematic research to develop and improve on Kegel's efforts and, as a result, the number of sufferers is rising dramatically. Given that these serious on-going health problems are directly caused by childbirth it is also extraordinary that there is still no concerted and effective programme of post-natal pelvic floor rehabilitation
• The media are in denial about the need for constant positive, accurate communication of the benefits of effective pelvic floor exercise

It is not that medical professionals are totally unaware of the issues and many experts recognise that there are problems. It is just that nothing positive seems to happen. For example, in 2002 an article in the British nursing press reported a study that showed that the link between childbirth and incontinence was not understood by most mothers, and that pelvic floor exercises were being poorly taught by health professionals. Over ten years later nothing has happened.

Chapter 2
What Arnold Kegel actually said

What did Arnold Kegel ever do for us?

Let us go back to the beginning and consider what Arnold Kegel actually did and why.

Arnold Kegel (1894 – 1981) identified the link between the diagnosis of urinary incontinence and prolapse, specifically following childbirth, and weakness, damage or atrophy in a muscle that we now refer to as The Pelvic Floor Muscle or Pubococcygeus (PC). Most crucially, he established that, with the correct exercise, this muscle could be restored to a healthy, well-toned state and the symptoms of incontinence and prolapse could be relieved.

The discovery that had even greater potential to make him famous was that these same exercises could restore sexual feeling and could enable women who had never achieved vaginal orgasm to experience one for the first time.

Shockingly, his research also pointed to the fact that surgery, offered to women as a solution to repair weak vaginal muscles, failed to work long-term.

In Kegel's seminal research paper published in 1948 (see Chapter 13) he noted *"Every physician has had occasion to observe that six months after a well performed vaginal repair with construction of a tight, long vaginal canal, the tissues, especially the perineum, will again become thin and weak".*

At the same time it was commonly accepted that suitable exercises could improve the function and tone of weak, stretched, atrophic muscles in all parts of the body and with this in mind, Kegel postulated that a specific form of active exercise could restore the various muscles of the pelvis.

His study over 18 years, focussed on the one muscle *"which has been largely overlooked by anatomists, obstetricians, and gynaecologists alike"* - the pubococcygeus. His conclusion was that the pubococcygeus is the most versatile muscle in the entire human body. It contributes to *"the support and sphincteric control of all pelvic viscera and is essential for maintaining the tone of other pelvic muscles, both smooth and striated."*

Most importantly he discovered that *"after having been stretched over a wider range than any other skeletal muscle (during childbirth!), the pubococcygeus can regain physiologic tension and, as we have demonstrated, it is able to recover its function after many years of disuse and partial atrophy."*

Arnold Kegel described the situation where the pubococcygeus (PC) muscle is found to be weak and atrophied as Genital Muscle Relaxation.

His research showed that Genital Muscle Relaxation, *"as manifested by urinary stress incontinence, cystocele, or prolapse of the uterus as well as certain types of lack of sexual appreciation, is always associated with - even if not directly due to - dysfunction of the pubococcygeus."*

His diagnosis was confirmed by the success of non-surgical treatment of these conditions, applying the general principles of muscle education and resistive exercise (exercise that involves squeezing against a resistance) to the pubococcygeus which he regarded as the pivotal structure of the pelvic musculature.

Identifying the right muscle

Kegel was clear in his observation that many women could not correctly identify and voluntarily contract the PC muscle and his study gave explicit guidelines as to how he could help train his patients to identify and contract their muscles at will.

It is still a fact today that many women, believing that they are 'doing their Kegel's', are actually engaging their abdominal muscles, the gluteus (buttock) muscles or the adductor muscles – their inner thighs. Recent clinical studies indicate that a third of women are unable to correctly identify and squeeze their PC muscle.

Kegel's machine

It was Kegel's search for a way to measure and improve the strength of the PC muscle that led to his development of the Perineometer – literally a meter or device for measuring the strength of the perineum.

Given the technologies available to him at the time, the Perineometer was a relatively simple, hydraulic apparatus consisting of a vaginal resistance chamber (like a big rubber squash ball) connected to a manometer (pressure gauge) calibrated from zero to 100 mm. of liquid mercury (Hg). The resistance chamber measured 2cm in diameter and 8cm in length, in line with the approximate dimensions of the normal vagina. It was designed to measure the pressure when the vagina was both resting and squeezed and the patient and doctor could read values off the vertical mercury column scale in much the same way as a doctor used to measures blood pressure. Arnold Kegel and his wife worked together for many years to assemble this equipment on the kitchen table – the forerunners of many entrepreneurs!

Luckily, modern women are not surrounded by a panoply of tubes and the benefits of the perineometer can be gained with much simpler, portable devices that perform most of the functions of Kegel's machine – see Chapter 9.

However, in modern medicine, the term 'perineometer' is now applied to electronic medical devices that are just designed purely to measure pressure. They do not provide the muscles with a feeling of resistance that can be squeezed against during exercise.

Trials with thousands of patients identified that good

muscle tone inside the vagina was shown by a 'resting' pressure of between 15 to 20 mm Hg.

If the pressure was as low as 10 mm Hg, Kegel realised that muscle tone was poor. When women with a normally developed pubococcygeus contracted the muscle (now known as a Kegel squeeze) there was a prompt increase in manometric reading to 20 mm Hg.

Kegel discovered that approximately 75% of patients could be trained how to squeeze the PC muscle after 10 to 20 minutes of instruction. In other instances, considerable patience was required and the instructions had to be repeated at weekly intervals, occasionally over a period of many months, before the patient learned to contract their PC muscle correctly.

One thing was clear. It was absolutely essential for the patient to be aware of their pubococcygeus muscle, and what it was doing when they squeezed, because unless they activated the muscle correctly there could be no improvement in their condition.

Visual Feedback

Kegel's trials with many women of all ages over many years confirmed that very few women who initially lacked an awareness of the function of the pubococcygeus would be able to continue correct contractions of this muscle at home after just one or two instruction sessions in the surgery or clinic. Since they were unable to coordinate their muscles through the usual reflexes, it was therefore necessary to establish a connection or feedback between contractions of the pubococcygeus and the brain. So, for the women, being able to see the movement of the mercury, proved vital to their understanding that they were squeezing correctly.

Today, this technique of learning a motor function through repetitive reinforcement is recognised as building the appropriate neural pathway between the brain and the local muscle. In the same way that people learn the actions of walking, typing or juggling in order to be able to do so without thinking, so it is often necessary to learn how to identify and squeeze the PC muscle. Some modern pelvic toning devices facilitate this learning.

Kegel's other landmark discovery was that learning the PC muscle squeeze was only one of the benefits of the Perineometer. The fact that patients could see how much the mercury moved meant they were immediately aware of any improvement and this was a significant boost to motivation. Kegel noted that without the ability to measure progress *"patients are apt to become discouraged"*. This is something of an understatement and a theme to which we will return.

Resistive Exercises

In addition to visual control, the Perineometer provided a means of contracting the perivaginal muscles against resistance.

Kegel noted, with a measure of understatement, that resistive exercises of this type have proved "most effective in all branches of muscle therapy for the correction of disuse atrophy and for restoration of normal function". He reported that resistive exercises *"strengthened the pubococcygeus in all its components, especially the minute end-fibres which, in genital relaxation, were usually atrophied."*

Supervision and monitoring

Despite his best efforts Kegel observed that about half of his patients who started their exercises correctly would soon lapse back into the old habit of using extraneous muscles instead of the pubococcygeus. Therefore, he recommended re-examination and repeated instruction at weekly intervals for one month, and thereafter as often as necessary to ensure correct use of the Perineometer.

Patients were encouraged to keep a progress chart to

monitor and record their improvement. It is therefore a fundamental principle of Kegel exercises that patients could record their ability to squeeze against progressively greater and greater pressures as measured by the Perineometer.

What were the benefits of Kegel Exercises?

Kegel's 1948 paper reported results on thousands of women and the objective and measurable improvements were impressive. He noted that in patients who exercised correctly and diligently, the following progressive changes would occur:

• *greater awareness of the pubococcygeus muscle and its function*
• *significantly improved muscle strength*
• *muscular contractions could be felt in areas of the vaginal walls where none could be demonstrated before*
• *development of the pubococcygeus so that weak and irregular contractions became strong and sustained.*
• *improvement in tone and texture of all muscle tissues of the pelvic floor*
• *an increased in muscle bulk of the pubococcygeus*
• *the vaginal canal became tighter and longer.*
• *previously flaccid vaginal walls improved in tone and firmness.*
• *bulging of the anterior vaginal wall (often diagnosed as 'moderate cystocele') becomes less pronounced.*
• *prolapse of the uterus, when present, was usually improved and in some instances the cervix ascended from being adjacent to the vaginal opening to as high as 5 to 7 cm. above the opening.*

All this could be achieved with the basic principles of effective training, visual feedback, resistive exercise and intense repetition over time.

It was a major factor that improvement could be

achieved very quickly and this, no doubt, increased motivation and compliance. In the case of stress incontinence Kegel reported:

"As some degree of awareness of function is initially present, the response to muscle education is prompt. Symptoms usually show improvement within two weeks after starting resistive exercises using the Perineometer. Lasting relief, however, depends on firm establishment of muscle reflexes and strengthening of muscular structures."

So why, oh why, were these principles not written in stone for all that followed?

A very modern perineometer

Over the last 15 years there has been a development in Progressive Resistance Vaginal Exercisers that meet all the principles that Kegel identified. Thanks to the internet, these are widely available and one model, the PelvicToner™, is also available on GP prescription throughout the UK.

In a US trial of this particular device doctors measured the physical improvement in muscle strength when resting and 'clenching' the pelvic floor.

"20 female patients with incontinence, bladder dysfunction and/or sexual dysfunction related to pelvic floor relaxation participated in a 16 week trial. An exercise programme using the device was taught and surveys were completed initially and at 8 weeks and study completion at 16 weeks. Pelvic tone pressure measurements at rest and during voluntary contraction effort were taken initially, and at 3, 8 and 16 weeks. 15 subjects completed the full course. Subjective improvement was noted by 73% of study subjects.

In the entire group overall mean resting pelvic muscle tone improved by 9.6%, while mean Kegel strength

14

increased by 28%. In the 7 of 15 subjects with improved resting tone, the mean increase was 38%. Thirteen of fifteen subjects (87%) had improved Kegel strength. Average pelvic tone measurements were increased at 3 weeks and continued to increase at 8 and 16 weeks. Subjective data collected by surveys revealed overall improvement in sexual satisfaction, bladder function and satisfaction with the program and use of the device. Thirteen (87%) of the participants indicated that they would continue the program and using the device on an ongoing basis."

These results confirm Kegel's original work but also confirm that a cheap, modern alternative to the original perineometer is available. And such is the effectiveness of these devices that users note significant improvement with just 5 to 10 minutes exercise each day.

Chapter 3
A little bit more anatomy

The Pubococcygeus Muscle

If we are going to discuss the problems caused by childbirth, and the role of exercise to effect improvement and recovery, then it is essential that we have a slightly better understanding of the bits of the body that we are talking about.

Kegel identified that the most important component of your pelvic floor is the pubococcygeus or PC muscle. In some contexts it is also referred to as the Love Muscle – but more of that later!

The pelvic floor or pelvic diaphragm is responsible for holding all the pelvic organs within the pelvis and, in fact, it supports the weight of your gut and all your internal organs. The muscles of the pelvic floor stretch like a hammock across the base of your pelvis, separating the pelvis from the perineum – the area between the anus and the vulva.

It is composed of several muscle groups in layers connecting at the front of the pelvic girdle (the pubis) and to the base of the spine (the coccyx) and to the bone structures on either side

The 'hammock' comprises the levator ani complex, coccygei muscles (of which the pubococcygeus is the most significant) and connective tissue.

The pelvic floor serves three principle functions:

• supports pelvic viscera and serves as the base of the abdomen supporting the bladder, intestines and uterus

- maintains continence and houses the neurovascular bundles and muscles that control urinary and anal sphincters
- facilitates childbirth and promotes foetal forward rotation through the pelvic girdle

The pubococcygeal muscles form a figure-of-eight stretching between the pubic bone at the front and your coccyx (tailbone) at the rear. The urethra and vagina pass through the front 'hole' and the rectum through the rear.

A healthy pelvic floor is crucial for every woman at all stages of her life. Bringing tone and vitality to this area will help live life to the full and protect you from many health problems. Exercising your pelvic floor you will help to strengthen the muscles which support the urethra, bladder, uterus and rectum. In turn this could dramatically alleviate urinary incontinence, support childbirth and discourage pelvic disease and menstrual problems.

Many women are aware of the need for pelvic floor exercises but few carry them out regularly and effectively. Today Kegel exercises, a pale imitation of what Kegel actually proposed, are often mentioned at ante-natal classes but they are rarely taught correctly and are soon forgotten. Only the disciples of yoga and Pilates are likely to more fully appreciate their benefits but even these rely on clenching and not squeezing against an external resistance. In yoga, the pelvic floor exercise, or mula bandha, is one of the fundamentals of core body strength.

Chapter 4
Exercises that really work

Fit for nothing!

It is often said that exercise is the answer to most health problems and that is particularly the case with the pelvic floor!

We all know that exercise is good for us and many of us have great intentions to do more – at least in the first few weeks of the New Year.

It also is heartening to see that over the past decade there has been a tremendous growth in public and private gyms and gym membership.

However, this surge of activity must be concentrated on a select minority because a recent study (March 2013) labelled British women the laziest and least fit in Europe. Our culture and lifestyle means that one in five admit they 'never do' any exercise. Compared to other European women, British women are much less likely to pursue individual or team sports into adult life.

One thing that is also all too apparent is that, in this modern age, everyone wants a quick fix. So, for some, taking a diet pill or a quick bit of surgery is much less effort than a workout.

This poses a challenge for everyone involved in trying to encourage greater levels of exercise, and a particular challenge for those promoting pelvic floor muscle exercises as the pelvic floor is literally 'out of sight, out of mind'.

An additional problem has grown from the fact that, successive generations have no faith in 'Kegel' exercises because they've *"tried them and they didn't work!"*

Even the knowledge that doing pelvic floor exercises really can improve your sex life, as many women have asserted, has failed to provide the necessary encouragement for women as a whole.

There is one reason for this. It is because the methods that have been promoted over the 65 years since Kegel introduced the world to 'his' exercise programme, bear absolutely no comparison to the rigour, intensity and duration he proposed.

Why would anyone waste their time on an exercise that does not seem to bring any benefit in any sort of reasonable time frame? The medical profession and the media must take responsibility for this by suggesting that *"eight to ten contractions, squeezing against thin air, three times a day, while you do the vacuuming or wait for a bus"* bears any relation to the three 20 minute sessions comprising 300 squeezes against resistance that Kegel found to work!

What is exercise?

At least one benefit of the growing gym culture is that more and more women are familiar with gym equipment and appreciate the benefits in terms of strength and body toning that they can achieve with cross-trainers, steppers, weight machines and barbells.

Every one of these pieces of equipment, and every physical exercise programme, involves the movement of muscles against a resistance. You only really exercise a muscle if you are lifting, pushing or squeezing something.

By definition:

* Exercise *"The act of using, employing, or exerting; systematic exertion of the body for the sake of health."*
* Exertion *"To strive, to use effort."*
* Effort *"An exertion of a physical or mental power, a strenuous attempt, an endeavour."*

19

Eight squeezes against thin air meets none of these definitions!

Most of us are aware of the sort of general fitness exercise programmes that are used in gyms, by Personal Trainers and recommended in magazines and newspapers. Many fitness experts talk about the 4 Rs:

Reinforcement

Muscles have to learn (or relearn) in order to function correctly. Even though many bodily functions seem to be involuntary – like walking – they only happen because initially you learn how to walk and the connection (the neural pathway between the brain and the muscle) has become imprinted. That pathway can fade with lack of practice as anyone who has had to relearn to walk after breaking a leg can testify.

Resistance

It is essential to make your muscles really work or exert effort so that you get the most from your exercise. The resistance aspect is the part of your exercise that builds strength. Resistance may be a weight you lift (including the weight of your own body or pushing against a pedal), or the resistance you have to squeeze against, such as hand grips or squeeze balls.

Repetition

This is all about doing enough exercise to exhaust your muscles and encourage the development of blood vessels and muscle tissue. Typically exercises for a particular muscle are performed in groups or sequences and described as 'sets' and 'reps' eg 3 x 10. What this means is that you perform a 'set' of 10 squeezes or lifts three times with a short rest between each set to allow the muscle to recover. When 3 x 10 feels too easy then you move up by increasing the number of repetitions and/or the number of sets eg to 4 x 10 or 3 x 15.

Regular

You must exercise regularly because, when you stop, the muscles lose their tone very quickly and can soon atrophy or die away. Again, those who have suffered a broken arm or leg will know just how quickly muscles can shrivel and fade to nothing. Just miss going to the gym for a few weeks and it is like starting over. The pelvic floor is especially susceptible because it gets so little exercise anyway. Search Google for 'vaginal atrophy' and you will find half a million references!

Performing lots of sets with relatively low weights/resistance is the way to develop muscle tone and definition – it's how flabby arms and bingo wings can be transformed into sleek, shapely limbs with no bulging biceps!

Performing fewer sets but with the maximum weight/resistance you can manage will build strength. This is the way to build real muscle bulk and develop athletic ability.

All exercises have these elements in varying degrees, even the cardiovascular exercises like running, cycling, rowing and cross-training that are designed to develop cardiovascular fitness and heart and lung function.

Every exercise programme follows these basic elements, that is, except the pelvic floor muscle exercises that are promoted in women's magazines and doctor's leaflets! Suggesting that women do 8 – 10 contractions against thin air is not exercise!

Why do you think that Kegel was so keen to constantly reiterate the need for 'resistive exercises'?

And more importantly, when, why and how did the need for resistance disappear from the development of the exercise programmes with which all women are so familiar and so frustrated? We will explore how this may have happened in Chapter 8 with a review of the clinical research.

Exercise correctly and effectively

So research shows that to do effective pelvic floor (Kegel) exercises you must use a device that provides a resistance for you to squeeze against and which provides the capability to increase the resistance so that, as you get stronger, you can work harder. These devices are readily available – see Chapter 9 - Progressive Resistance Vaginal Exercisers.

A second benefit of using such a device is to help you confidently identify your PC muscle and give feedback to confirm that you are squeezing the right muscle.

Chapter 5
Better sex after babies

Towards a better sex life

If you think that your sex life is fantastic and that you couldn't possibly achieve more orgasms, more easily then you do not need to read this chapter. However, pelvic floor weakness, or Genital Muscle Relaxation, following childbirth or the menopause has been found to reduce the intimate contact during intercourse and it is common for both partners to report that it becomes much more difficult to achieve orgasm through vaginal intercourse alone.

There is also good evidence that healthy, well-toned muscles have a much better blood supply and more nerve endings and women with a strong pelvic floor muscle report more vaginal orgasms of greater frequency and greater intensity.

If sexual intimacy causes problems, this can impact on the whole relationship so it is obviously an important matter to address and resolve.

In his 1948 study, Kegel described a normal vagina thus: *"In the normal vagina, the canal is tight and the tissues offer a degree of resistance from all directions. The walls close in around the finger as it is inserted, moved about, or withdrawn."*

Reports of women not being able to retain tampons and vaginal weights are worryingly and surprisingly commonplace. It is also not normal for the vaginal cavity to fill on immersion in water. Situations where you must stand in the bath to 'drain' before exiting do not reflect normal muscle tension.

Is my vagina too big?

It is very clear that the issue of 'vaginal tightness' is one that occupies the minds of many women and, probably, many couples. Searching discussion groups, blogs and advice pages on the internet indicates that a question taxing many women is "Is my vagina too big?" A Google search with the words 'loose vagina' brings up over 25 million responses!

And it is not as if the medical profession are unaware of the problem – or the possibilities it presents!

Writing in the UK Sunday Times in June 2011, Lois Rogers wrote:

"Many women see delivering a baby as an emotional high point and could not imagine missing a second of agonising pain, despite the fact that, according to the Lancet, up to one in three of them will afterwards suffer some form of incontinence, and up to one in six some form of sexual dysfunction. In the 266-page NICE document are figures of 64% of women suffering sexual problems six months after childbirth, and a 21% risk of incontinence. An average figure of almost £7,000 is given for lifetime treatment of incontinence, and that is still assuming everyone dies by the age of 80. And fewer than two in three of the women affected actually see a doctor. No treatment at all is suggested for sexual problems."

The article went on to quote a female obstetrician who rather tactlessly – and graphically –remarked:

"You do see a lot of British women with vaginas you could drive a bus up. I think a lot of them just accept that forgoing sexual pleasure is the price they have to pay for having children."

Type 'cosmetic surgery vaginal tightening' into Google and you get 3.5 million results with pages of companies offering surgery that can cost over £10,000.

In an article on the subject in October 2011 Marie Myung-Ok Lee, writing in the UK newspaper The Guardian, wrote:

"Designer vagina surgery is big business: according to the American Society for Aesthetic Plastic Surgery, in 2009 female consumers spent an estimated $6.8m (£4.4m) on these procedures (the figure counts only plastic surgeons, not gynaecologists). Its popularity is rising in the UK, too.... figures released this year show that plastic surgery company The Harley Medical Group received more than 5,000 inquiries about cosmetic gynaecology in 2010, 65% of them for labial reduction, the rest for tightening and reshaping."

The role of the pelvic floor

In some texts the PC or vaginal muscle is also called the Love Muscle or Fire Muscle and this highlights the role of the pelvic floor in sex. Various sources say that during orgasm the vaginal muscle contracts repeatedly every 0.8secs

One thing that can be said for certain is that women who believe they have a strong pelvic floor report better orgasms than women who acknowledge that they have a weak pelvic floor. (Source: 5000 respondents www.orgasmsurvey.com).

The question is – why?

We cannot say whether Kegel's lengthy research was initially motivated by a desire to improve the sex lives of women but, given the cultural conditions of the time, this would probably be unlikely. However, we can be certain that he took note of the subjective feedback of his patients. For those working in this field, even today, it is common to hear a woman recently versed in the finer points of real

Kegel exercises with the appropriate device to exclaim *"Wow! Doesn't it improve your sex life!"*

So it is no surprise that just four years after publishing his major work Kegel was reporting on the sexual functions of the Pubococcygeus.

"Observations in [more than 3,000 women,] both parous* and nulliparous*..., ranging in age from 16 to 74 years, have led to the conclusion that sexual feeling within the vagina is closely related to muscle tone, and can be improved through muscle education and resistive exercise."

"78 of 123 women complaining explicitly of sexual deficits achieved orgasm following the training".

Arnold H. Kegel "Sexual Functions of the Pubococcygeus Muscle" Western Journal of Surgery, Obstetrics & Gynecology, 60, pp. 521-524, 1952

*having given birth and not having given birth

It is perhaps also relevant to remind ourselves that it is about this time (1950) that the German Ernst Grafenberg claimed to have found the mythical G-spot and the role of the clitoris became the subject of intense research.

Whilst many men have spent the ensuing years frantically trying to rediscover this elusive location, the links between various parts of the female anatomy and the ability to improve the orgasmic experience seemed to get lost in the mists of time.

It is also difficult to assess the impact of the feminist movement and the debates about the relative roles of the clitoris and the vagina in sexual politics (eg Anna Koedt, The Myth of the Vaginal Orgasm, 1970). Some at the time were arguing that the vagina was just a 'receptacle for male gratification' and played no part in female enjoyment. Given that environment it would be hard to argue that the sex benefits of pelvic floor exercises had any relevance at the time.

Then, in 2008, further light was shed on the perineum

when Italian scientist Emmanuele Jannini carried out extensive research using ultrasound and claimed to have found a 'thickening of the tissue' in the vaginal wall in women who could achieve vaginal orgasm. He noted that:

"the vast majority of women do not have this 'thickening' which explains why they cannot find their G-spot and do not get vaginal orgasms."

It is difficult to say with any clarity whether this increases or diminishes our understanding of the problem, but this would appear to be the same tissue that Arnold Kegel referred to when he identified a direct link between a well-developed pelvic floor muscle (ie a thickening of the muscle wall) and the ability to have a vaginal orgasm.

Kegel didn't have access to ultrasound but he used palpation and physically measured the strength that women had in their pelvic floor and stated categorically that there seemed to be a link between strong muscle tone and the ability to achieve orgasm.

Exercise for a better sex life

Surprisingly there seems to have been little research in recent years that has progressed the thinking on the subject.

Whilst most of the pelvic floor exercise devices on the market claim that they will 'enhance the sex life' there is little objective assessment.

As the manufacturer of one pelvic toning device my company carried out a survey of women who were taught how to exercise correctly, following Kegel's principles:

"Before using the PelvicToner™ progressive resistance vaginal exerciser only a third of women said they 'often' or 'always' achieved a vaginal orgasm during penetrative sex. 43% said 'never' or 'rarely'.

After using the PelvicToner the results were 'never' or 'rarely' ZERO. Those saying 'often' or 'always' 75%"

This is definitely an area that needs more objective and scientific research. One thing is certain. The whole subject of sexual satisfaction and the ability to achieve orgasm, of any kind, is an incredibly complex one and factors such as health, physical health, emotional state, tiredness etc must be taken into account.

We are also in an era when the major pharmaceutical companies are attempting to define Female Sexual Dysfunction as a disease and to develop pharmacological drugs to cure it.

In the circumstances, it is incumbent on those with any relevant knowledge on these matters to share it with the population at large. If sexual enjoyment can be impaired because muscles are weak or atrophied, and if the damage can be repaired with simple exercises, then it is for the greater good that this information and the correct techniques are shared. And it must be hoped that a greater awareness that effective exercise can restore or improve your sex life should be seen as a significant motivation to exercise on a regular basis.

Chapter 6
Other embarrassing health issues

The long term impact of childbirth

Childbirth can have a very traumatic effect on the pelvic floor so it is important, if you can, to do everything possible to strengthen your pelvic floor before you even get pregnant. In the same way that it is proven that dietary supplements such as folic acid should be taken in advance of pregnancy, so you should plan to make your pelvic floor as healthy and as strong as possible.

Weak pelvic floor muscles can lead to poor muscle action during labour and childbirth making delivery difficult and lengthening recovery to full health and fitness.

A strong pelvic floor muscle can enable a woman to carry a baby more comfortably during pregnancy and will help both the mother and baby during labour and delivery.

Stimulating blood flow in the pelvic area after childbirth quickens recovery from any stitches or episiotomy (an incision made to the perineum between the vagina and anus to ease delivery of a baby).

Women who have had or plan to have a Caesarean delivery also need to strengthen their pelvic floor muscles as it is the gravitational pressure of pregnancy that weakens the muscles not just the physical event of birth.

Having said that, it is very much the process of natural childbirth that causes the greatest damage to the pelvic floor and the problem seems to be exacerbated by forceps delivery.

A recent study (Obstetrics & Gynecology, November 2012 - Volume 1200) assessed mothers 6-11 years after childbirth. It demonstrated conclusively that pelvic muscle strength is significantly reduced over a long period of time by vaginal birth and further reduced by forceps delivery.

The study recommended that secondary prevention of pelvic floor disorders may be accomplished by targeting women with a history of vaginal birth [perhaps a proactive post-natal pelvic floor rehabilitation programme that this author has been advocating for many years!]

The study author Victoria L. Handa, Professor of Obstetrics and Gynecology at Johns Hopkins University said:

"In prior research, we demonstrated that pelvic floor disorders including incontinence and pelvic organ prolapse were significantly more common among women who delivered by vaginal versus caesarean birth. We also demonstrated that pelvic floor disorders were strongly associated with forceps delivery. However, the biological mechanisms underlying these associations are unknown. In the present study, we test the hypothesis that vaginal childbirth is associated with pelvic muscle weakness, the rationale being that pelvic muscle weakness is thought to contribute to the development of pelvic floor disorders. It has never before been shown that pelvic muscle weakness is a risk factor for the development of pelvic floor disorders.

Our results reveal long-term differences in pelvic muscle strength between women who have experienced vaginal birth and those who have delivered by caesarean. While these findings do not prove that delivery mode causes subsequent changes in pelvic muscle function, we speculate that impairment of pelvic muscle function may be a critical factor underlying the observed association between mode of delivery and pelvic floor disorders."

She had obviously never read the research papers by Arnold Kegel, but this study was first modern attempt to assess the impact of childbirth on long-term pelvic muscle strength and function.

The Menopause

As women enter the menopausal years (35-54) their oestrogen levels decline. Oestrogen is a female hormone that readies the body for childbirth and is no longer produced in large amounts once menstruation ends. The muscles and tissues of the vagina are particularly sensitive to oestrogen levels circulating in the blood and a decrease in oestrogen can cause changes in vaginal tissue leading to atrophy, and a decrease in vaginal lubrication.

This loss of adequate lubrication can cause painful intercourse and increases the chance of injury and infection to the vagina or bladder.

The reduction in oestrogen accelerates muscle atrophy leading directly to Genital Muscle Relaxation.

For women who may have lived with slight problems of incontinence or prolapse following childbirth this natural degeneration of the muscle can have a profound and long-term effect if no action is taken to reverse the underlying cause.

Urinary Incontinence

Contrary to popular myth, urinary incontinence is NOT a normal part of ageing. It affects women of all ages, and especially new mums. Between a third and a half of all new mums report incontinence problems and the situation can then become much worse following the menopause when atrophy of the vaginal muscles accelerates with the decline of oestrogen. By the time women reach their mid50s half will experience incontinence some, or all, of the time.

Because of the personal and embarrassing nature of the problem, and the belief that no help is available, many women do not report their symptoms to their doctors and few discuss their problems with family, friends and even their partners.

Research indicates that women will suffer, on average, for up to 7 years before consulting their doctor. Yet today's health care professionals offer a number of treatment options to improve bladder control, such as pelvic muscle exercises, biofeedback, bladder training, drugs and even pelvic surgery. This subject is addressed in far more detail in the Chapter 7.

There are two types of urinary incontinence: stress incontinence and urge incontinence.

In stress incontinence, urine leaks out occasionally when doing such things as coughing, sneezing, lifting, or exercising. It can be just a mildly irritating inconvenience resulting in a damp patch in the groin which many women manage with pantyliners or an incontinence pad. But, without treatment, the problem can get much worse and can necessitate a complete rethink of one's social activities.

Doctors still recommend pelvic floor exercises as the first approach to urinary stress incontinence and research over many years still claims that pelvic floor exercises can cure 80% or more of suitable cases.

The focus of this book is very much on ensuring that the pelvic floor (Kegel) exercises you do are as effective as possible and follow the guiding principles recommended by Arnold Kegel.

Urge incontinence means that a woman is unable to hold her urine when there is a strong need or urge to urinate. Women that suffer from urge incontinence also tend to have more urinary tract infections and skin problems than other women.

The risk of urge incontinence is especially high during or after pregnancy, following childbirth, during and after menopause, in cases of obesity and cigarette smoking, following surgery, hysterectomy, radiation therapy to the pelvis; in cases of diabetes, Parkinson's Disease, back injury, cerebral vascular accident and dementia.

Urge incontinence is more likely to be treated with bladder training and pharmaceutical intervention but pelvic floor exercises can play a role by increasing muscle control and giving greater confidence of the bladder functions.

Incontinence is a significant worldwide problem:

• Over 200 million women suffer from incontinence world -wide
• It is estimated that between 5 and 7 million women in the UK suffered incontinence in the past year
• Stress incontinence affects one in three to half of new mums

Historic research suggested that between a quarter and a third of all menstrual pads sold were used to self-treat incontinence. However, in recent years a whole new industry has emerged to satisfy the worldwide trend for fashionable, continuous- wear incontinence pads

Incontinence and menstrual pads only address the symptoms, not the root cause of the problem, and also pose major environmental issues.

Genital or Pelvic Organ Prolapse

Approximately 30%-40% of women develop some presentation of vaginal prolapse in their lifetime, usually following childbirth (especially multiple births), menopause (due to the lack of oestrogen), or a hysterectomy (the removal of a key element of anatomical support).

Most women who develop this condition are older than 40 years of age but the problems usually have their origins much earlier in life. Many women who develop symptoms of a vaginal prolapse do not seek medical help because of embarrassment, limited understanding of the symptoms and effects or other reasons.

Some women who develop a vaginal prolapse do not even immediately experience symptoms which can include: discomfort when bearing down to have a bowel movement; occasional, slight vaginal bleeding; vaginal infections; or loss of bladder or bowel control.

Pelvic floor exercises are recommended for the treatment of mild to moderate prolapse and to supplement other treatments. Whilst this book is very much focussed on the role of effective exercise it cannot be stressed enough that if you have symptoms that may suggest a prolapse then you must seek medical help. By all means follow the guidance contained within this book if your doctor suggests exercise or if you wish to try some self-help in conjunction with medical treatment, but be guided by your doctor.

The network of muscles, ligaments, and skin in and around a woman's vagina acts as a complex support structure that holds pelvic organs and tissues in place. This support network includes the skin and muscles of the vagina walls (a network of tissues called the fascia). Various parts of this support system may eventually weaken or break, causing a common condition called vaginal prolapse - a condition in which structures such as the uterus, rectum, bladder, urethra, small bowel, or the vagina itself may begin to prolapse, or fall out of their normal positions. Without medical treatment or surgery, these structures may eventually prolapse farther and farther into the vagina or even through the vaginal opening if their support weakens enough.

The most common symptom of all types of vaginal prolapse is the sensation that tissues or structures in the vagina are out of place. Some women describe the feeling as "something coming down" or as a dragging sensation. This may involve a protrusion or pressure in the area of the sensation. Generally, the more advanced the prolapse, the more severe the symptoms. The symptoms that result from vaginal prolapse commonly affect sexual function as well as bodily functions such as urination and defecation.

Cystocele (prolapse of the bladder, bladder drop)
This can occur when the front wall of the vagina (pubocervical fascia) prolapses. As a result, the bladder may prolapse into the vagina. When this condition occurs, the urethra usually prolapses as well. A urethral prolapse is also called a urethrocele. When both the bladder and

urethra prolapse, this condition is known as a cystourethrocele. Urinary stress incontinence (urine leakage during coughing, sneezing, exercise) is a common symptom of this condition.

Rectocele (prolapse of the rectum) –

This type of vaginal prolapse involves a prolapse of the back wall of the vagina (rectovaginal fascia). When this wall weakens, the rectal wall pushes against the vaginal wall, creating a bulge. This bulge may become especially noticeable during bowel movements.

Vaginal vault prolapse

This type of prolapse may occur following a hysterectomy, which involves the removal of the uterus. Because the uterus provides support for the top of the vagina, this condition is common after a hysterectomy, with upwards of 10% of women developing a vaginal vault prolapse after undergoing a hysterectomy.

In vaginal vault prolapse, the top of the vagina gradually falls toward the vaginal opening. This may cause the walls of the vagina to weaken as well. Eventually, the top of the vagina may protrude out of the body through the vaginal opening, effectively turning the vagina inside out. A vaginal vault prolapse often accompanies an enterocele.

Prolapsed uterus (womb)

This involves a weakening of a group of ligaments called the uterosacral ligaments at the top of the vagina. This causes the uterus to fall, which commonly causes both the front and back walls of the vagina to weaken as well. This can present in four stages:

• First-degree prolapse - The uterus droops into the upper portion of the vagina.
• Second-degree prolapse - The uterus falls into the lower part of the vagina.
• Third-degree prolapse - The cervix, which is located

at the bottom of the uterus, sags to the vaginal opening and may protrude outside the body.

- Fourth-degree prolapse - The entire uterus protrudes entirely outside the vagina.

Prolapse treatment

Most vaginal prolapses gradually worsen and can only be fully corrected with surgery. However, the type of treatment that is appropriate to treat a vaginal prolapse depends on factors such as the cause and severity of the prolapse, whether the woman is sexually active, and the woman's treatment preference.

Nonsurgical options may be most appropriate for women who are not sexually active, cannot undergo surgery because of medical reasons, or experience few or no symptoms associated with the condition.

Oestrogen replacement therapy may be used to help the body strengthen the muscles in and around the vagina.

Pelvic floor exercises are used to tighten the muscles of the pelvic floor. Pelvic floor exercises might be used to treat mild-to-moderate cases of vaginal prolapse or to supplement other treatments for prolapses that are more serious.

Chapter 7
Doctor, why don't you help?

What can your Doctor do for you?

The one thing your doctor or midwife will probably not offer you is an effective post-natal pelvic floor rehabilitation programme. This would help restore your pelvic floor muscle to a more healthy state, prevent the onset of urinary stress incontinence and restore muscle tone to prevent prolapse.

This is in contrast to other administrations, notably France, where every new mother is given vouchers for a ten week programme of physiotherapy. But don't get too excited! The original objective of La rééducation périnéale après accouchement (perineal retraining after childbirth), first introduced after the First World War, was not based on the medical needs of mothers but to restore their 'honeymoon freshness' so that mums could quickly get back to the business of making love and making more babies!

The National Institute for Health and Clinical Excellence (NICE) is the organisation that sets the standards for all treatments across the UK National Health Service (NHS). There are guidelines for post-natal care in the UK (NICE CG37 2006) that say:

"Women with involuntary leakage of a small volume of urine should be taught pelvic floor exercises. "

There is no other mention of the pelvic floor in these guidelines so the methodology is left to the Clinical Guidelines for the treatment of incontinence – see below.

Discussion groups and other researches I have undertaken confirm the impression that many women believe that post-natal care is too 'baby-centric' and that there is too little real help and guidance for the new mother. Or for older women come to that. A wealth of research confirms that most new mothers believe that urinary incontinence is either unusual, and that their condition is uncommon, or that it is usual and that nothing can be done about it. These beliefs seem to be engendered by poor education and information systems and an inadequate response from the medical profession at all levels from the midwife to the GP.

The problem is significantly compounded because of the taboo nature of incontinence so that there is no willingness to discuss the issue before or after birth and in a medical or social context. Whatever the background, the NHS does have options and offers exercise, drugs and surgery. The focus of this book is on the exercise aspects.

NICE Guidelines

The National Institute for Health and Clinical Excellence (NICE) published clinical guidelines for the treatment of urinary incontinence in women (CG40) in October 2006. The process of reviewing these guidelines began in 2012 and is on-going - see below.

At this point it is worth revisiting the fundamental principles of Kegel's exercises:

• Muscle training and learning with the development of the neural pathway from brain to pelvic floor
• Feedback to confirm to the user that the correct muscles are being engaged
• An intense programme of daily resistive exercise ie exercises where you squeeze against a resistance
• Progressive resistance so that the user can measure and monitor improvement over time and increase the resistance in line with their improving strength

NICE CG40 recommended pelvic floor exercises in the conservative management of stress incontinence saying:

"A trial of supervised pelvic floor muscle training of at least 3 months' duration should be offered as first-line treatment to women with stress or mixed UI.
There is good evidence that daily pelvic floor muscle training continued for 3 months is a safe and effective treatment for stress and mixed UI. "

The word supervised is stressed and the role of a specially trained person such as a physiotherapist is fundamental to the NICE recommendation. Without the active on-going involvement of a specially trained nurse or physiotherapist to assess you and monitor your progress you are not receiving the appropriate level of treatment.

The assessment process would normally include a determination of the condition of the pelvic floor muscle. The scale used most commonly by physiotherapists is the Modified Oxford Scale (MOS). This is a 6-point scale described as: 0 =no contraction, 1 = flicker, 2 = weak, 3 = moderate (with lift), 4 = good (with lift), 5 = strong (with lift). This involves putting a finger into the vagina and assessing the 'squeeze' that the patient can bring to bear.

The NICE Guidelines then go on to specify what the exercise should involve:

"First-line treatment for stress or mixed UI should be pelvic floor muscle training (PFMT) lasting at least 3 months.
• Digitally assess pelvic floor muscle contraction before PFMT.
• PFMT should consist of at least eight contractions, three times a day.
• If PFMT is beneficial, continue an exercise programme.
• During PFMT, do not routinely use:
• electrical stimulation; consider it and/or biofeedback

in women who cannot actively contract their pelvic floor muscles
• biofeedback using perineometry or pelvic floor electromyography"

Extract from NICE CG40 Full Guidelines App E pp161 -162

Biofeedback is a mechanism or indicator that confirms that a biological or physiological function, such as a squeeze, is being performed correctly.

The UK Chartered Society of Physiotherapy offers a slightly more robust set of exercises saying:

"build up your routine, aiming towards doing this three times a day:

• Squeeze and lift as strongly as you can. Hold for ten seconds. Relax ten seconds. Repeat ten times
• Follow with ten fast squeezes. Squeeze and lift as hard and as briskly as you can and then let go completely"

However, these exercise regimes clearly lack the level of exertion that Kegel recommended and this must have a major influence on the outcomes. Few physiotherapists expect to see much improvement in three months with the NHS approach which is in stark contrast to the results reported by Kegel and his experience that resistive training could bring objective improvement of symptoms in two weeks.

At what point, and by what method, this treatment could evolve from Kegel's original proposals is unclear and we will explore this further in the next chapter.

Notwithstanding that, pelvic floor muscle training (PFMT) is not a cheap option for the NHS as the following 2006 figures from NICE demonstrate:

"Costings are based on treatment being undertaken by a senior 1 grade women's health physiotherapist in a

40

hospital physiotherapy department. There are a total of six sessions with the therapist. The initial session lasts 1 hour; subsequent sessions last half an hour.

Labour costs - Contact time with patient: (1 × 1) + (5 × 0.5) = 3.5 hours. Unit cost: £37 per hour. Labour cost: £37 × 3.5 = £129.50

Consumables Cost Total £1.50

Total cost for PFMT: £131 (£94 to £168) 2006 prices"

What you can expect

Given these costs it is not surprising that few women presenting to their GP with symptoms caused by pelvic floor weakness are even referred to physiotherapy, notwithstanding the fact that physiotherapists are a very scarce resource and most hospitals have significant backlogs for physiotherapy treatment.

A survey of GP practices in 2012 showed that remarkably few (less than half) were actually aware of the detail of the NICE Guidelines and that the recommended first line treatment was a three month programme of supervised pelvic floor muscle training.

Only 20% of the practices responding claimed to send patients to physiotherapy for examination and treatment.

In 62% of cases women seeking help or advice because of pelvic floor related problems were given a leaflet. There are no clinical trials or clinical evidence to support or condone this course of action. It does not take a genius to see the link between this practice and the fact that some 7 million women in the UK still suffer from stress incontinence!

There is clearly a need for a much more robust response to pelvic floor problems because, as has been previously noted, clinical evidence suggests that a third of women are unable to identify their pelvic floor muscle and squeeze it on demand (0 or 'no contraction' on the Oxford Scale).

It is also well known that compliance with any form of exercise programme is low, and if there are no clear and early indications to link the exercises with a measurable improvement in muscle tone or strength then there is little motivation to continue with the exercise. How many women truly complete their exercise programme with daily exercises for three months?

Asking women to complete a three month programme based on ineffectual exercises, with no guidance or direction, and a system that offers no feedback that they are even engaging the correct muscle, and that brings no significant improvement, is not a recipe for success. It is therefore no surprise that few women undertake pelvic floor exercises of any kind or with any regularity.

Furthermore, imploring women to do 'their Kegel's' while they vacuum or wait for the bus hardly gives the exercises the focus or gravitas they deserve.

It was reading about current practises, and realising just how many women are left to suffer unnecessarily, that led me to develop a medical device which would address these issues. The PelvicToner™ Progressive Resistance Vaginal Exerciser is currently the only clinically proven pelvic toning device on NHS Prescription (see Chapter 9).

Many GPs are now prescribing the PelvicToner and many hospital physiotherapy departments have welcomed this 'new technology'. However, there are still those who regard any change to the status quo with an almost Luddite zeal!

As the PelvicToner, used unsupervised, has been shown to be as effective as supervised pelvic floor muscle training, it is surprising that it has not been adopted more widely – especially as it costs just one tenth of the alternative supervised treatment.

For those who do not benefit from exercise, there are over 150 operative procedures for stress incontinence. One of the most common operations is the insertion of a supportive tape (TVT Tension-free Vaginal Tape). There are also a number of drug therapies. The reader should carry out her own research to more fully understand these options.

In the absence of any real improvement from NHS exercises most women with incontinence rely on absorbent pads to manage their problem until matters get really serious and they will then go under the knife. Kegel's observations, anecdotal evidence and the number of class action legal cases reported on the internet suggest that even that is not always wholly satisfactory.

The 2012 Review of NICE Guidelines

In 2012 NICE began a review of the CG40 Guidelines and I hoped that this would include a review of the new techniques and devices that had become available since 2006 – including the PelvicToner™ progressive resistance vaginal exerciser . One would have expected that with a clinically proven pelvic toning device available on GP prescription it would be considered as a significant alternative for first line treatment in primary care.

Despite intense lobbying of NICE, the decision was made that the scope of the review would not include a fresh look at lifestyle interventions, physical therapies and non-therapeutic interventions. Instead, the review concentrates exclusively on pharmacological and surgical interventions and, as a result, a great opportunity has been missed to reintroduce real Kegel exercises.

A radical review is necessary

There is clearly an issue with pelvic floor exercises as far as the medical profession is concerned and there seems to be an element of Catch-22 in addressing the problem.

There seems to be one school of thought that there is no point in pushing the point because women will not do what they are told! A physiotherapist summed up the dilemma concisely saying:

"I don't see that the issue is that the number of

squeezes has been reduced - it's that women don't comply with even 10 squeezes."

The lack of compliance with any exercise routine is always going to be difficult but the challenge is even greater if the patient has issues with identifying their pelvic floor in the first place and then the exercises are of such low level that there is no perceived, or even expected, improvement within two or three months.

Kegel reported that his patients were more highly motivated to continue with their exercise because they could physically see that they were improving day to day and within a couple of weeks they had better control of their bladder. With similar results, there is no doubt that women would be more motivated to progress with their 21st Century treatment.

There is then the matter that, despite clear clinical guidelines for what constitutes 'best practice', patients are being failed in their primary care, ie by GP surgeries.

Writing in 2010 Professor Marcus Drake of the Bristol Urology Institute said:

"Primary care does not provide supervised pelvic floor exercises except in rare cases. The vast majority of women are handed a leaflet and not examined. Supervised Pelvic Floor Exercises are known to be better than that rather poor service. Supervised means that women are actively taught the Pelvic Floor contraction by a highly trained healthcare professional (and hence it is expensive)."

With all the historical evidence that pelvic floor exercises can be effective we need to understand why the exercise programmes recommended to women today are so inadequate, how these programmes were developed ignoring the principles that described an effective best practice, and why there has not been systematic research to improve the effectiveness of exercise using the best modern techniques and methods.

Chapter 8
Where did it all go wrong?

Why are Kegel's principles ignored?

The author is not the first to ask this fundamental question and may not be the last – as long as someone somewhere acknowledges that non-invasive exercise can be preferable to the surgical alternatives.

Dr John D. Perry writing in 1988 noted that:

"The medical establishment is polarized about the value of Kegel's Exercises:

On the one hand "patient advocates", such as nurses and physical therapists, insist that (l) anyone can learn to do them, (2) everyone should learn to do them, and (3) they each know the one "correct" way to teach them.

On the other hand, most urologists and gynaecologists only politely smile at the mention of Kegel's legacy, knowing full well that, sooner or later, almost every incontinent person will eventually submit to a surgical procedure or urological medication."

(Source: The Bastardization of Dr Kegel's Exercises, John D Perry 1988)

The historical situation is perhaps most succinctly summarised by one of the leading lights in incontinence research. Professor Kari Bo writing in Evidence-Based Physical Therapy for the Pelvic Floor: Bridging Science and Clinical Practice (2007) says:

"In 1948 Kegel was the first to report pelvic floor muscle training (PFMT) to be effective in the treatment of female

urinary incontinence. In spite of his reports of cure rates of over 84%, surgery soon became the first choice of treatment and not until the 1980s was there renewed interest for conservative treatment. This new interest for conservative treatment may have developed because of higher awareness among women regarding incontinence and health and fitness activities, cost of surgery and morbidity, complications and relapses reported after surgical procedures.

Although several consensus statements based on systematic reviews have recommended conservative treatment and especially PFMT as the first choice of treatment for urinary incontinence, many surgeons still seem to regard minimally invasive surgery a better first-line option than PFMT."

A lack of clinical research

This very long gap between Kegel's original announcements and the new enthusiasm for non-surgical intervention in the mid-1980s also explains the why there is such a gap in the clinical research.

There are a number of comprehensive reviews published over the last 7 – 8 years that consider all the published research for exercise. Given the scale of the problem, and the potential for an effective non-surgical treatment, it is surprising that most reviews only reference around 50 clinical studies.

Throughout the research and the reviews there is consensus that supervised PFMT is more effective than standard postnatal care – whatever that may entail!

Although Kegel's 1948 paper is cited in practically every published clinical research paper it is notable that there does not seem to have been any attempt to repeat Kegel's studies, there does not seem to be any research to prove or disprove his claim that resistive exercise was essential and there is little evidence of any systematic research to determine the optimum amount of daily exercise.

How many squeezes?

What is perhaps even more surprising is that there is little indication of when and how the rationale for 8, 10 or 20 squeezes emerged. In the absence of any evidence it must be assumed that the decision was arbitrary and that few subsequent researchers saw the need question the methodology adopted in previous research.

In The 3rd International Consultation on Incontinence 2005 (Professor Paul Abrams et al) there is a clue in the paragraph that states:

"It is not clear what the most effective parameters are; clinicians and researchers should refer to exercise physiology literature to provide biological rationale for their choice of training parameters. PFMT parameters can be selected based on the aim(s) of the treatment, eg muscle strength, endurance, co-ordination and function. Therefore programs might comprise small numbers of maximal or near maximal contractions held for short periods, repeat once or more daily, at least three times a week (suggests strength training) and/or a moderate number of, daily, sub-maximal contractions held for long periods (suggests endurance training)."

In contrast, in a paper entitled 'The status of pelvic floor muscle training for women' (Canadian Urological Association Journal Dec 2010) the authors write:

"To improve general muscle strength and power, sedentary, sick or elderly individuals are recommended to perform 1 to 2 sets of 8 to 12 preset exercise repetitions at a frequency of 2 to 3 times per week".

This paper does not suggest a regime for a fit healthy individual but notes that a review of protocols reveals a range of recommendations for pelvic floor muscle contractions that extend from 5 to 200 per day.

It concludes by saying that the *"optimal"* protocol for PFMT is *"still elusive"* and that *"physical therapists should discuss all the different elements that underlie a patient's pelvic floor weakness and dysfunction; this would allow the physical therapists to design an individual program for the patient."*

So our conclusion must be that there is no real rationale for 8, 10 or 20 squeezes and someone just guessed.

The use of resistance

John D Perry (Source: The Bastardization of Dr Kegel's Exercises, 1988) observed that:

"Unfortunately, history found it easier to transmit Kegel's words than his device (the perineometer). The latter was marketed for many years by Kegel and his wife, who assembled the components - literally - on their kitchen table.

Mrs Kegel diligently continued the practice for three more years following his death. The gradual decline of the device may be reflected in its inappropriately stable price: from 1947 to 1979, it always sold for the same $39.95 at which it was first introduced.

Lacking ordinary commercial incentives, the medical equipment industry lost interest in the perineometer. Lacking his perineometer, medical personnel were forced to improvise on his methods. The results of trying to teach Kegel's exercise without his measuring device have been less than impressive "

Perhaps the greater pressure came with the development of pharmaceutical and surgical solutions and the financial power these large companies were able to bring to bear to fund clinical trials and to persuade the medical profession to use and promote their new techniques.

In contrast, many of the pelvic floor exercise devices we now see in the market have their origins in small entrepreneurial companies that lack the financial stature to fund the necessary research, gain respect and credibility with the medical profession and to break into the market. Many are small-scale companies operating on the same scale as Kegel did himself. That doesn't mean they are not trying!

A glimmer of hope

There has, however, been one clinical study in the recent past where the PelvicToner™ progressive resistance vaginal exerciser was compared to the NICE standard protocol for supervised PFMT. Titled "A randomised controlled trial of the PelvicToner Device in female stress urinary incontinence" the results of the trial have been published in the British Journal of Urology International (Jan 2010) and the International Urogynecology Journal (May 2013).

In the trial, randomly selected subjects were only allowed to use the device at a minimum level of resistance and minimal activity. They were instructed to carry out a standardised PFMT regime consisting of five 'quick' and five 'slow' (sustained), high intensity pelvic floor contractions daily over a 16 week period.

It has to be stressed that the trial did not evaluate the PelvicToner being used in line with the manufacturer's directions which recommend the progressive increase of both repetitions and resistance from 3 x 10 repetitions at the lowest resistance up to 3 x 50 at the highest level with the patient progressing as fast and as far as they feel able based on their subjective assessment of improvement.

Nonetheless, the study concluded that the PelvicToner was as good as supervised PFMT (even without the element of progressive resistance) and "aided women to identify their pelvic floor confidently. It is a safe and well tolerated adjunct to PFMT, which increases patient choice and may promote subsequent compliance and sustained efficacy."

Looking forward

In summary it would be fair to say that the exercise programmes currently recommended do not seem to have the hard evidence to support them. There may be a view that they 'work' or are better than nothing but that is not really a sound scientific or clinical basis. Without a systematic analysis of the problem, for example, are 20 squeezes better than 8, 100 better than 50, 200 better than 100, then one can only infer that the selection of any specific number of squeezes is purely arbitrary.

1. The idea that eight simple muscle contractions repeated several times a day can even be called 'exercise' is also questionable.

Kegel's assertion was that exercise should take the form of three 20 minute sessions daily (sometimes translated as 300 squeezes per session) against resistance and with feedback being a fundamental requirement. Until someone can prove that there is an alternative that works better, this should be established and remain as the Gold Standard. Therefore it would seem logical to conduct clinical trials to confirm that Kegel's theories still hold good and to actually compare the outcomes with the current best practice.

There is clearly a feeling within the medical community that there is no point suggesting more than eight or 20 or 50 squeezes because women would not do them anyway. This comes down to issues of compliance and feedback and would be addressed by implementing exercises of sufficient rigour that they demonstrated to the user that improvement was being achieved, that the effort was worthwhile.

However, with the use of Progressive Resistance Vaginal Exercisers that feedback and reinforcement of the benefits is demonstrated very easily – as one very satisfied customer of the PelvicToner reported: *"When I started I could only manage 20 squeezes with the minimum resistance. Now I can do 3 sets of 50 squeezes with a much higher resistance. And I feel tighter inside!"*

The exercise regimes that are currently recommended lack the feedback, the resistance and the intensity that Kegel proved were critical. These crucial elements are not present in the recommended exercise regimes but they are in those associated with Progressive Resistance Vaginal Exercisers and there must be more trials to prove the worth of these devices. Especially as they offer a much cheaper as well as a more effective solution to the NHS.

Chapter 9
Self-help solutions

Caveat emptor – buyer beware

By now you will hopefully appreciate that the lack of effective preventative treatment has created a situation where there are many millions of women suffering with problems associated with pelvic floor weakness.

This has created a huge business opportunity and stimulated an enormous growth in appliances, devices and remedies that purport to offer cures and treatments. The growth of the internet may have modernised the sales and distribution channels but the market is still awash with 'snake oil' sellers and quacks.

This book is not the place for a complete analysis of all the products on offer or a comprehensive listing of sellers and prices. There is certainly a very good case for a comparative, systematic, clinical evaluation of many of these products to help women separate the wheat from the chaff.

My observations are based upon my own researches and discussions with many hundreds of women over the last ten years. You are left to draw your own conclusions.

Progressive Resistance Pelvic Floor (Vaginal) Exercisers

It is worth reminding ourselves again of the fundamental principles of Kegel's exercises:
- Muscle training and learning with the development of the neural pathway from brain to pelvic floor

- Feedback to confirm to the user that the muscles are being engaged
- An intense programme of daily resistive exercise
- Progressive resistance so that the user can measure and monitor improvement over time and increase the resistive force in line with their improving strength

This is the only group of devices that have been specifically designed to address these principles and to concentrate on the progressive resistance aspect. At the time of writing there are three products available on the internet:

The Gyneflex™ - A system of moulded, flexible plastic V-shapes that offer six levels of resistance. US designed and manufactured. The complete set sells for around £116.

The Kegelmaster™ - A spring based device shaped like a dildo (obviously). The four springs offer multiple levels of resistance. US designed and manufactured. The Kegelmaster sells for £50 - £60.

The PelvicToner™ - A spring based device similar in shape and principle to the Kegelmaster. Offers 5 levels of resistance. Developed and manufactured in the UK by the author. The PelvicToner sells for around £30 but is the only clinically proven pelvic toning device on GP prescription in the UK which means that it is available for £7.85 (current prescription charge) and free to new mothers in possession of a Maternity Exemption Certificate and to the over 60s.

All these devices appear to be capable of matching Kegel's achievements in that *"symptoms usually show improvement within two weeks after starting resistive exercises"*.

Their design, and the very specific way in which a resistance can be applied to the exercise process, makes these devices far more effective than Kegel's Perineometer and most users achieve significant improvements with just 5 to 10 minutes exercise each day.

Indicators and trainers

These are usually soft small spherical or ovoid devices that you insert into the vagina so that you can 'learn' the correct muscle to squeeze and confirm that you are squeezing correctly. They often have a protruding arm that remains outside the vagina and the correct squeeze will cause the arm to move up and down.

They are a useful training device and are often used in hospital physiotherapy departments. They help you identify the correct muscles and help train your muscles and develop the neural pathway but they lack the resistance capabilities to make your exercises truly beneficial over time.

They can be purchase from around £15.

Electro-stimulation devices

You will be familiar with the advertisements for a 'twitching' belt that would tone your abdominal muscles and give you a washboard stomach. Many saw this as a product perfect for those who lacked the will and motivation to actually do some exercise. They were probably correct.

Well, the population with a weak pelvic floor is at least a great as that with flabby abs and the 'vibration' has now moved inside with a small vaginal probe that stimulates the vaginal muscles to contract repeatedly at great speed.

These machines use the TENS principle (Transcutaneous Electrical Nerve Stimulation) which was originally developed to treat pain. When used to stimulate muscles electric current is used to cause muscles to twitch involuntarily.

Unfortunately the real benefit of these devices can best be summed up by imagining a scenario of Victoria Pendleton, Sir Chris Hoy and Sir Bradley Wiggins training for the Olympics by hurtling around the cycle track on a moped. *"No pain, no gain"* – in the words of Jane Fonda!

Electro-stimulation devices do not address any of the key principles identified by Arnold Kegel. The experience is purely passive so there is no active exercise, no training of the muscles and no development of the neural pathways. There is no resistance so whilst the muscles may develop a degree of muscle tone through repeated twitching, there is no possibility of them actually increasing their strength.

The situation with these devices is perhaps best summed up by leading urologist Professor Marcus Drake writing in the British Journal of Urology International:

"These alternatives are not recommended by NICE and are not universally advocated by clinicians as they have yet to produce sufficient evidence of efficacy."

Having said that, electro-stimulation does have a role and is used in physiotherapy clinics where the patient is completely unable to identify and to squeeze the pelvic floor muscle.

The devices are marketed for between £50 and £600 – finance plans available!

Vaginal cones, weights and balls

Variations are also referred to as jade eggs, Venus balls, Ben Wa balls and orgasm balls, and the name indicates that these are more designed for erotic stimulation. However, there are 'clinical' versions that have been used for many years and some users claim improvement – but compared to what?

In clinical trials, vaginal weights were the least effective in the comparison of weights, electro-stimulation and 'NHS style' pelvic floor exercises and only 20% of users saw an improvement compared to the 'best' result – pelvic floor exercises – where 50% saw improvement. They are not recommended by NICE.

There is plenty of chat about theses weights and balls on the internet eg *"unless you are extremely tight they do have a tendency to fall out of place rather easy"* and they should come with a health warning: Do not use when standing on ceramic floor tiles!"

They are widely available in shops and on the web from around £20 to £100 subject to the material used and extravagance of the packaging.

The bizarre

Not every manufacturer bothers to read the medical literature with the result that there are 'pelvic floor exercisers' that go nowhere near the pelvic floor and, for purely anatomical reasons, could not live up to their claims.

Typical of these is a Y shaped plastic device squeezed between the thighs "Slip this exerciser between your upper thighs, squeeze your muscles against the resistance of the device for a few minutes, twice daily, and you'll start to feel the benefit in your buttocks and thighs too."

It may be good for the adductor muscles but Kegel would be spinning in his grave!

Chapter 10
Embarrassment for some is a goldmine for others

Who is soaking up your hard-earned cash?

There was a time, not long ago, when the term 'incontinence' conjured up pictures of the geriatric ward and old folks at the ends of their lives and in a state where the lack of bladder and bowel control was just one more indignity to suffer.

Oh, how it has all changed. For the industry with the most to gain, incontinence is now a subject for prime time TV advertising and continence products are a fashion accessory for the glamorous girl who has everything – literally.

Incontinence management is still a serious matter and many millions rely on a plethora of products that most of us are glad to be totally ignorant of. We may be aware of the existence of adult nappies (diapers) and special absorbent underwear but we dread the need to delve further into this murky world of bags and tubes.

But most of these products meet a need for particular types of incontinence that are caused mostly by age, infirmity and disability. This is not the condition that Kegel was addressing all those years ago.

The embarrassing leaks that are experienced by so many women from the new, young mother to the fit healthy 70 year old are caused by muscle weakness. Instead of manifesting as a permanent, chronic condition, stress incontinence leaks can occur unexpectedly – but especially when you cough, sneeze, laugh, exercise, dance etc. The fear factor with stress incontinence is that it can occur at any time and particularly when you are enjoying yourself in a social environment.

There are no outward signs that you are a sufferer, just a damp feeling when you do.

This presents the really big opportunity for the manufacturers of absorbent pads. Instead of catering for a market that requires the use of a pad for perhaps five to seven days each month and between the years of 13 and 50, here is a whole new market that requires protection every day of the month from the birth of your first child until you visit that great lavatory in the sky.

Just think of the potential!

A huge growing market

You probably cannot even come close to guessing how much money is involved.

Writing in the quaintly termed Nonwovens Industry Review March 2012, the editor Karen McIntyre, penned an article entitled "Adult Incontinence: Not Your Grandmother's Market ". She wrote:

"With an estimated 200 million people affected globally, adult incontinence is becoming more widespread as older populations continue to represent a larger demographic segment around the world. An overwhelming majority of sufferers are women—approximately 75-80% - and, while it is usually considered a concern of the elderly, more younger people are afflicted.

In fact, a recent survey, conducted by Cotton Incorporated of 115 million known sufferers in the US, found that the fastest growing population in this market is obese African-American women between the ages of 20 and 30.

Therefore, companies doing business in the adult incontinence space have to juggle a number of different needs. There are light incontinence sufferers who usually get away with using feminine hygiene products to mask their condition; stress incontinence sufferers, who use a combination of products depending on the day and heavier incontinence sufferers who want products they can use discretely while maintaining the active lifestyles they crave. Then, of course, there is the institutional market catering to the extremely old or sick and bedridden.

Add to this the stigma surrounding the market, with many sufferers buying alternative products to avoid the shame associated with incontinence, and these manufacturers have their hands full.

However, the rewards are worth the aggravation as this is one market within hygiene that is predicted to grow worldwide.

Unlike the disposable baby diaper market—which is characterized by low birth rates and high penetration rates in developed markets and manufacturers have to look at emerging areas for growth—adult incontinence has plenty of room to grow in places like the US and Western Europe where active seniors and even younger sufferers will pay top dollar for products that are effective."

How did it all start?

It is easy to see why this market has developed.

When the US National Association for Continence surveyed consumers in the late 90s, about 60% of consumers said that they used some type of disposable liner or pad or underwear. It is noteworthy that at that time over a quarter of all women with incontinence said they used sanitary pads (napkins) and nearly a fifth of all women used tissues, paper towels, or toilet paper in lieu of any specially designed absorbent product.

For a forward looking manufacturer this is the sweet sound of cash tills.

In 2001 Kimberly Clark stated that "the US adult incontinence retail/home care market had grown 3.1% to reach $594 million in 2000 - a figure that did not reflect institutional sales to hospitals and nursing homes". They were projecting that in the year 2005, the US retail and institutional sales of the manufacturer would reach $2.1 billion and global sales would hit $5.8 billion. In 2001 Kimberly Clark's share of the adult incontinence market was 52.4%. These figures now seem like a gross underestimate.

In 2012 SCA, the Swedish manufacturer of TENA pads, estimated that the global annual market for incontinence products is valued at some SEK 70bn (£7bn), and is growing at about 5% annually, with Europe accounting for approximately 40% of the total market, closely followed by Asia-Pacific and the US.

It's about quality of life

The vice president communications of incontinence care Europe for SCA was quoted as saying:

"The baby boomers are entering their golden years and they carry high expectations from their products for good quality of life. At the same time, the financial crisis combined with the growing elderly demographics has put pressure on the healthcare systems globally, which directly affects healthcare products. We must focus not only on developing high functioning products but also on economical solutions for the players."

One of the key questions that is not addressed is whether the perpetual purchase of incontinence pads is as economical for the consumer as a simple, effective cure using Kegel exercise.

SCA is a great example of a company that has recognised the potential. TENA is the market leader in the UK and the aforementioned industry review noted that:

"SCA has made acquisitions in Taiwan, Turkey and Brazil and has worked hard to promote its TENA brand of adult incontinence items in North America".

In 2012 SCA appointed top global advertising agency TBWA\London to handle its £40 million global advertising account for its TENA range of which an estimated £4 million is being spent in the UK market. In addition to high profile TV advertising, TENA is promoted with extensive magazine advertising, sales promotion and sampling and even sponsorship of 'timeless classics' on daytime TV.

Industry analysis reported recently that "Widened and improved product offerings are strengthening the position of the incontinence market" and this is perfectly illustrated by the TENA product range. To meet the requirements of the one in two women that SCA estimate experience 'light bladder weakness' TENA offers fifteen product and pack variants of TENA Lady and TENA Lights.

"The protective underwear product that we have launched provides mobile users to have complete discretion and security," says SCA. "Incontinence solutions must target not only functional absorption requirements but also address emotional needs as well in providing dignity, self-confidence and improved quality of life."

Those in need of reassurance and a better quality of life could easily spend £150 or more a year which over just 40 years is an expenditure equivalent to the purchase of a small car.

A focus on customer care

As with all new markets, the industry has recognised that the consumer has to be convinced of the need for a purpose-designed product and requires help to make 'the correct purchase'. All the major manufacturers invest heavily in customer care and sampling designed, like their advertising, to portray the need for incontinence pads as perfectly natural and normal. Again, Kegel would be spinning in his grave!

In the early days Kimberly-Clark estimated that 80% of

first-time users of incontinence products would be unsure which product to buy and could spend around £100 trying to find the right product. To help them, their Depend brand team created no- and low-cost sample kits that included various products, information booklets and special offer coupons.

In addition to making its customers feel comfortable, Kimberly-Clark has worked hard to develop new products catering for a new type of adult incontinence user, one that looks at the years beyond 65 and retirement differently than previous generations. And, with this demographic in the US expected to grow from 40 million to 55 million between now and 2020, Kimberly-Clark, like SCA, sees category growth in incontinence is crucial.

And again, like SCA, Kimberly-Clark has targeted the new market of younger fashion-conscious women. They even invented another new medical condition in the process!

The new hourglass-shaped Poise pads are especially designed to meet the needs of women with light bladder leakage. These pads *"have first-of-a-kind "pink lace" graphics and are packed in an attractive pouch, for a feminine look and feel. The unique contoured shape of the new Poise innovation curves around the legs, enhancing the fit around the natural curves of a woman's body."*

No-one is saying that incontinence pads are not relevant or important. It is just that if the underlying problem was cured then managing the symptoms would not become a lifetime issue.

Light bladder leakage, light bladder weakness, light adult incontinence, stress incontinence – they are all the same and collectively they present a huge business opportunity

Chapter 11
The role for the media

Why is the media important?

You may wonder what role the media could possibly have in the treatment and cure of stress incontinence. But in fact, it is hard to under-estimate the part that they have played and could play in the brave new world.

It is difficult to decide what is worse – disseminating inaccurate information and guidance or failing to communicate anything at all.

One thing is clear, and that is that in the current environment the media have a more critical role than any other party.

In their online helpline the UK NHS acknowledge that almost half (45%) of all people with incontinence wait at least five years before they get help,

Research in the US reported a similar statistic saying that:

"women with urinary incontinence typically wait almost seven years before seeking help from a medical professional ... if they seek help at all! In fact, only 50% of women with urinary incontinence do seek help. The rest simply suffer in silence and cope with the symptoms as best they can."

Women suffering from incontinence may not be seeking help from their doctor but you can be sure that they are seeking out information or absorbing the material presented in the magazines and newspapers that they read.

The most ridiculous part of the above statistics is there are so many forms of help available for women's urinary incontinence, from simple lifestyle changes to minimally-invasive surgeries with high rates of success. So why do so many women wait so long to seek professional help for their urinary incontinence, or refuse to seek help at all? And what should the media do to better fulfil their role.

Relevant information

One aspect could be the reaction of the medical profession when patients do pluck up the courage to ask for help and opinions of the medical profession which the patient may hold. Many discussion groups confirm that post-natal care is seen as very baby-centric and that the problems of the mother are a lower priority.

Many mothers complain that doctors do not take the initiative to ask the right questions and raise the more embarrassing questions in an appropriate way. Many complain of closed questions ("Are you doing your Kegels?") without appropriate guidance as to how they should be done correctly (if only) and without mention of the long-term consequences of doing nothing.

Then there is the effectiveness of the response. As we have discussed in a previous chapter, the majority of surgeries merely pass on a leaflet with no real guidance or instruction and leave the poor sufferer to get on with it. This is very wrong on so many levels.

The media can play a very substantial role here by trying to correct misperceptions about the problems, emphasising the universal nature of stress incontinence and reinforcing the fact that it is a totally normal and common problem that can it can be quickly and effectively cured in most cases.

Embarrassment

Even when a sufferer finally plucks up the courage to seek advice women's urinary incontinence tops the list of health conditions that ladies feel most embarrassed about discussing with their doctors. As a result of wanting to avoid a red-faced discussion, 50% of these women are prepared to suffer almost seven years of urinary urgency, frequency, and leakage before gathering up the courage to ask for help. The other half would rather suffer the symptoms than have "the talk" about urinary incontinence with their doctors.

Medical research in Sweden found a similar picture. Women aged 23-51 years with persistent urinary incontinence took part in a telephone interview survey. Three-quarters of the women with a long-term problem had not sought help. The most common reason given was that the disorder was considered a minor problem, which they felt they could cope with on their own. When women did finally consult professional help they did so because they were afraid of the odour of urine and that they perceived the leakage as shameful and embarrassing.

It is not just the sufferers who succumb to the embarrassment of discussing one of the last great taboo subjects. Just ask any manufacturer of products related to incontinence and they will tell you that they meet a wall of indifference from journalists and health editors.

One national newspaper editor told me:

"It's not a subject that people want to read about over their cornflakes".

That doesn't seem to be an issue when we are inundated with techniques to improve our sex lives and achieve better orgasms – even if few of the articles mention the role that pelvic floor exercises could play!

A moving target

The final problem is one of frequency. Talk to the more enlightened health editor of any mainstream women's magazine or national newspaper and the response you may get is:

"We covered stress incontinence three years ago and there are greater priorities".

It may be that the editors have just not realised the scale of the problem, but one small calculation indicates why there are few greater priorities.

In the UK there are around just over 700,000 births each year, that is around 60,000 each month or 15,000 each week. All the available research suggests that around a third of new mothers go on to suffer from stress incontinence – 5000 women every week. Many more will suffer from prolapse and many, if not all, could benefit from help to restore their sex lives.

The issue does not have a three yearly cycle. Every day of every month of every year women are discovering the symptoms that are caused by pelvic floor weakness.

The print media and the internet are a primary source for accurate and meaningful information and, in the absence of direct and appropriate medical advice, they are the place to which most women will turn for help. It is therefore essential that the subject matter is treated with the importance that it deserves.

Chapter 12
What could we do better?

What do we know?

Let us just consider some of the 'givens'.

We know that stress incontinence is a very significant problem for millions of women and that it is caused by pelvic floor weakness usually following childbirth and the menopause, but obesity and general fitness are other significant factors.

We know that prolapse is also a very serious problem with the same basic causes.

There is clear evidence that sexual satisfaction can be affected for the same reasons.

We know that awareness of the causes and effects of these problems is poorly understood because the information available is generally inadequate.

There is overwhelming evidence that regular, effective pelvic floor exercises can provide objective cure for all this conditions, in the vast majority of cases, but that the exercises recommended by the medical profession and the media fail to meet the rigour necessary with the result that outcomes are generally poor and compliance is low.

What is the problem?

There seem to be four main issues:

Firstly, and for reasons that just cannot be explained, the method of rigorous, resistive pelvic floor exercise that was clinically proven by Arnold Kegel with trials on thousands of women over decades, became transmuted into a pale imitation that required barely one hundredth the time and no physical effort.

Secondly, there has been no consistent, accurate education of women at large to emphasise the link between the pelvic floor and on-going health issues. There has been no consistence education to make women aware of the consequences of childbirth and the menopause, and to improve their understanding of the causes and effects that both can inflict on the pelvic floor.

Thirdly, there has been, and is, no effective guidance or training for the techniques of pelvic floor exercise, as recommended by Kegel, that could bring enormous relief and cure to so many both in a self-help and medical context.

Finally, for many years there was not a device that could emulate the key role played by Kegel's perineometer.

We have the technology

With the death of Arnold Kegel the key component of his treatment, the perineometer, soon disappeared off the scene. At the time the technology was more limited and there was clearly little incentive for manufacturers to develop more effective and economic devices.

Doctors and manufacturers certainly saw that there was a major opportunity to develop surgical interventions. Over recent years the pharmaceutical industry has begun to realise that this is a huge and profitable market and now there are a plethora of drugs to address the symptoms of stress incontinence and sexual dysfunction. The manufacturers of absorbent pads did not need any encouragement.

The entrepreneurial climate of the last fifteen years has led to the emergence of many small companies attracted to the self-help market by the scale of the problem, the potential of the internet to promote and distribute products, and the lack of effective mainstream solutions.

Finding a way to make pelvic floor exercises more relevant has been the focus of much ingenuity and, whilst not all of these inventions could really claim proven effectiveness, it has increased the general amount of web chatter and offered information and hope to many.

There are a handful of products, the Progressive Resistance Vaginal Exercisers, that do meet the fundamental principles identified by Kegel and one of them can truly claim to be clinically proven. These devices have proven to be effective, they are simple to use, they are much cheaper than other treatment options and they are certainly cheap enough to be made universally available.

A brave new world

What can women expect and what should they demand in this brave new world?

Certainly the answer must be "Something much better than we have at the moment!"

Going back to the four main issues identified above, it would not be overly ambitious to hope that we can look forward to a more positive approach to the use of pelvic floor exercise and to do this four things need to happen:

1. Better education in the need for pelvic floor exercises and the long-term problems that pelvic floor weakness can cause
2. Clinical trials to confirm that the exercise regime proposed by Arnold Kegel delivers better outcomes for women than the current best practice.
3. Proper training in exercise techniques using Progressive Resistance Vaginal Exercisers that reflect the rigour and principles that Arnold Kegel proved were necessary
4. A pro-active response from the medical profession to ensure that all women are offered the very best advice and help starting with an all-encompassing programme of Post Natal Pelvic Floor Rehabilitation designed to address the underlying health problem before it becomes an issue for most women.

Kegel's New Legacy

At the present time Kegel's Legacy is nothing really to be proud of. He is associated with an exercise regime that bears no resemblance to his research, few women are truly aware of its relevance and even fewer practice it on a regular basis.

It is abundantly clear to some that Kegel's principles still hold true and that they are even more relevant today than they were 65 years ago.

In 2013 there are devices that fulfil the role of the perioneometer, the potential for effective communication is greater and more universal than Kegel could ever have imagined, and the need is huge.

With a collective will there is no doubt that Kegel will have a worthwhile legacy as the man who determined that millions of women need not suffer in silence.

It is hoped that this book will help initiate informed debate and make many more women aware of the potential that exists to release them from one of the last great taboos. From this day onwards nothing is taboo!

If you have been suffering from stress incontinence, prolapse or poor sex because you have neglected your pelvic floor then now go forward with confidence. With the information in this book you should be able to practice your pelvic floor exercises with confidence and success.

Do something positive for yourself, and then tell your friends!

Chapter 13
Arnold Kegel – Unexpurgated

A Nonsurgical Method of Increasing the Tone of Sphincters and their Supporting Structures

Arnold H. Kegel, M.D., F.A.C.S. Assistant Professor of Gynecology University of Southern California School of Medicine

Source: Arnold H. Kegel, MD, FACS. Stress Incontinence and Genital Relaxation. CIBA Clinical Symposia, Feb-Mar 1952, Vol. 4, No. 2, pages 35-52.

Every physician has had occasion to observe that six months after a well performed vaginal repair with construction of a tight, long vaginal canal, the tissues, especially the perineum, will again become thin and weak. It was this repeated observation which first aroused the author's interest in the physiology of the pelvic musculature.

Everyone agrees that suitable exercises will improve the function and tone of weak stretched, atrophic muscles. A point in fact is the correction of faulty posture. Why then would it not be possible to restore through active exercise the normal anatomic relationships of pelvic structures, since they depend so largely for their support on various muscle groups?

In the study of this problem, which we have carried out over a period of 18 years, we have become greatly interested in one muscle, the functional importance of which has been largely overlooked by anatomists, obstetricians, and gynecologists alike - the pubococcygeus.

This muscle, when observed in emaciated cadavers, is in such a state atrophy that it would seem to be capable of little function.

The surgeon who operates from below encounters only the more superficial muscles of the vulvar outlet and argental diaphragm. This is true also of prophylactic episiotomy. Similarly, operations from above rarely include the pubococcygeus. It is for these reasons that the importance of this muscle has not been fully recognized.

Attention has been focused on the pubococcygeus by the studies of Barry J. Anson with Curtis and McVay who, in dissections of young female cadavers, demonstrated for the first time that the pubococcygeus gives off innumerable fibers which interdigitate and insert themselves into the intrinsic musculature of the proximal urethra, middle third of the vagina and rectum.

Our own study in the dissecting room, in surgery, and in animal experiments, as well as observations of the effect of exercise in several thousand patients, has led us to conclude that the pubococcygeus is the most versatile muscle in the entire human body. It contributes to the support and sphincteric control of all pelvic viscera and is essential for maintaining the tone of other pelvic muscles, both smooth and striated.

After having been stretched over a wider range than any other skeletal muscle, the pubococcygeus can regain physiologic tension and, as we have demonstrated, it is able to recover its function after many years of disuse and partial atrophy.

Palpation demonstrates that in a normal pelvis with the viscera in their normal position, the pubococcygeus and all of its components are well developed. However, when genital relaxation has occurred, this muscle is found to be weak and atrophied.

Genital muscle relaxation, as manifested by urinary stress incontinence, cystocele, or prolapse of the uterus as well as certain types of lack of sexual appreciation, is always associated with - even if not directly due to-

72

dysfunction of the pubococcygeus. This fact has been borne out by the success of non-surgical treatment of these conditions, applying the general principles of muscle education and resistive exercise to the pubococcygeus as the pivotal structure of the pelvic musculature.

The fasciae are not discussed here for the reason that, whether injured or intact, they depend upon their muscular attachments for nourishment, viability, tone and tensile strength. When grossly disrupted they remain a surgical problem.

Diagnosis

A firm vaginal canal, well closed to a high level, indicates normal development of the interdigitating fibers of the pubococcygeus. Loss of tone and prolapse of the vaginal walls, as is found in genital relaxation, signify weakening and thinning of these minute branchings.

The musculature of the middle third of the vagina is readily palpated by means of the index finger introduced up to about the second joint, or 3 to 5 cm beyond the introits.

In the normal vagina, the canal is tight and the tissues offer a degree of resistance from all directions. The walls close in around the finger as it is inserted, moved about, or withdrawn. Upon palpation, the walls of the middle third of the normal vagina feel firm throughout, and adjacent tissues give the impression of depth and good tone because the terminal fibers of the pubococcygeus are well developed and are attached to the intrinsic tissues of the vagina over a wide area.

In genital muscle relaxation on the other hand, the findings are decidedly different. Whether the introitus is gaping or tight, the vaginal canal in its middle third is short and roomy in all directions. The walls offer little resistance to the palpating finger and feel thin and loose, as if detached from the surrounding structures. The tissues between the palpating finger and the symphysis or rami of the ospubis are thin, tender, and of poor quality. From this it can be concluded that the muscular structures in the perivaginal regions are atrophied, particularly the terminal fibers of the pubococcygeus.

Vaginal examination as described up to this point differs little from the usual technique practiced for the past hundred years. The physical status of the perivaginal tissues has thus been ascertained, but the cause of weakness and atrophy has not been determined. To this end it is necessary to investigate the functional status of the supportive and sphincteric muscles of the pelvic outlet, especially of the pubococcygeus.

The first step in the examination for function is to observe whether by voluntary effort the patient is able to retract, draw up, or draw in the perineum. Next, the index finger is introduced into the middle third of the vagina, and the patient requested to contract upon it. Normal patients will respond immediately, and a firm grip upon the finger is felt over a wide area. Others, lacking awareness of function of the pubococcygeus, will not respond to the instruction and will often state that they did not know that it was possible to contract vaginal muscles. It is in this group of patients that palpation demonstrates the atrophy of disuse.

The digital method of ascertaining the presence of contractions of the perivaginal muscles should be supplemented by the diagnostic use of the Perineometer. With this instrument, strength of contractions in the middle third of the vagina as well as the width of the contracting area can be measured and a progress chart of record kept to follow the results of therapy.

The Perineometer is a simple, pneumatic apparatus consisting of a vaginal resistance chamber connected with a manometer calibrated from zero to 100 mm. Hg. The resistance chamber measures 2 cm. in diameter and 8 cm. in length and is formed by a cylindrical rubber diaphragm stretched to a specific tension between two flanges on a metal stem. The vaginal parts of the Perineometer conforms to the approximate dimensions of the normal vagina and is so designed that pressure over a wide area will result in higher readings than pressure of identical strength applied to a narrow area. The vaginal chamber is compressible, without significant compensatory expansion.

The specifications of this simple apparatus were established after 18 years of experimentation with more than 30 different types of instruments. Only in rare cases, when the vagina has been greatly shortened through surgical intervention or radium therapy, will it be found necessary to reduce the size of the vaginal chamber of the instrument.

When the resistance chamber is introduced, a slight rise on the scale of the manometer will be noted even before the patient exerts any effort. This represents the static pressure which in a normal vagina amounts to 15 to 20 mm. Hg. and indicates good muscle tone and tissue resistance over a wide area.

In genital relaxation, muscle tone is poor and tissue resistance is limited to a narrow area. Consequently, in such cases the initial pressure is low, about 10 mm. Hg.

Contractions of a normally developed pubococcygeus are registered by a prompt increase in manometric reading to 20 mm. Hg. or more above the initial static pressure. Lack of awareness of function and degrees of atrophy of the pubococcygeus are reflected by a small or almost imperceptible increase in pressure, usually less than 5 mm. Hg. Intermediate readings may be obtained in patients having awareness of function but only a narrow, poorly developed or partially atrophied pubococcygeus muscle. In measuring function of the pubococcygeus, it must be made certain that the patient is not using extraneous muscles, such as those of the abdominal, gluteal, or introital regions.

Therapy

Physiologic therapy of genital muscle relaxation is divided into two phases or steps: (1) specific muscle education and (2) resistive exercises of the pubococcygeus and its visceral extensions.

Specific Muscle Education

The first and most important step in therapy is muscle education. This is directed toward establishing adequate awareness of function of the pubococcygeus, which is the pivot of all supportive and sphincteric structures of the pelvis.

At the first office visit, approximately one third of all patients will be unable to contract the pubococcygeus voluntarily, or to only a questionable degree. When such is the case, palpation is continued until the examiner finds among the contiguous muscles, one which is under the patient's control. With this as a starting point, contractions of the contiguous muscle are continued and varied until the pubococcygeus itself is affected by such muscular movements.

The contractility of the pubococcygeus can be determined most readily in its anterior portion, where the fibers converge toward attachment to the os pubis, and posteriorly near the coccyx. In order to demonstrate contractions near the pubis, the postero-inferior margin of the symphysis is identified with the index finger, which is inserted only to the second joint.

The tip of the finger is passed laterally from the midline for about 0.5 to 1.0 cm. until the tendinous medial margin of the pubococcygeus is encountered; the margin is then followed downward for a short distance, approximately to the level of the urethra. At this point, contractions of the pubococcygeus, if present, are felt as a tensing of its medial margin, which may feel like a thin sheath, or it may be as broad as thick as a finger.

The pubococcygeus is palpated for function on both sides. Occasionally, unilateral impairment due to injury is revealed. In identifying the pubococcygeus, it should be remembered that congenital variations occur in its aponeurotic attachments.

Posterior contractions of the pubococcygeus are identified by inserting the finger deeply into the vagina or rectum. When palpating in the midline, the pubococcygeus can be felt near its attachment to the coccyx. With the finger in contact with the muscle, the patient is requested to contract it. Normally it will be noted that the posterior portion of the muscle has the ability to rise upward for a distance of 2 to 4 cm.

If there is lack of awareness of function of the pubococcygeus, no such voluntary action can be elicited. The patient is then requested to draw up or draw in the anus as though checking a bowel movement. Pressure may also be applied with the tip of the finger to aid the patient in identifying and contracting the pubococcygeus. If no response is forthcoming, pressure is increased to the point of discomfort, and the patient instructed to pull the muscle against the finger. In obstinate cases, reflex contractions may be produced by pricking the skin lateral to the anus. Repetition of any such action of the pubococcygeus for several minutes will usually enable the patient to continue the same contractions through voluntary effort. To make certain that the contractions elicited are those of the pubococcygeus and not of the iliococcygeus, they are followed anteriorly until they can be felt as tensing of the medial margins of the muscle at the level of the urethra.

Under the guidance of the physician, the patient who initially lacked awareness of function of the pubococcygeus has at this point learned that the muscle can be contracted voluntarily.

Since therapeutic results can be expected only from frequent repetition of active contractions of the pubococcygeus, these efforts are now described in terms of muscular functions of which the patient is cognizant.

With his finger on the medial margin of the pubococcygeus at the level of the urethra, the physician instructs the patient to (1) squeeze the vaginal muscles upon the palpating finger; (2) draw up or draw in the perineum; (3) contract or draw up the rectum as though checking a bowel movement; (4) contract as though interrupting the flow of urine while voiding.

The examiner makes sure that while performing these movements the patient is actually contracting the pubococcygeus and not merely muscles around the orifices. It must be emphasized that woman with poor function of the pubococcygeus have all their lives compensated for this deficiency by depending for support upon the fasciae and the more superficial muscles.

If the pubococcygeus is not functioning the following will be observed:

When an effort is made to draw up or draw in the perineum, no actual retraction occurs. Instead there is a tightening of the gluteal muscles together with sphincteric action which is confined to the introital group of muscles, including the bulbocavernosus, the transverse perinei, and the superficial pillars of the levator ani.

In the effort to contract as though to stop the flow of urine, only a slight twitching of the meatus of the urethra is observed, without retraction of the urethra itself or of the vaginal tissues overlying it. These shallow, superficial contractions are in themselves of no value in the prevention and treatment of genital relaxation and urinary stress incontinence. When contracting as though to check a bowel movement, the action is limited to puckering of the anus, and no retraction of the anus is observed.

The patient may be permitted to repeat these superficial contractions temporarily, but she is urged to try to transfer them to a higher level of the pelvic outlet, until contractions of the pubococcygeus muscle are felt by the palpating finger. Approximately 75 percent of patients will respond after 10 to 20 minutes of instruction. In other instances, considerable patience is required and the instructions must be repeated at weekly intervals, occasionally over a period of many months, before the patient learns to contract the pubococcygeus. In exceptional cases, the attempt to establish awareness of function fails completely. This is usually due to concomitant lesions of the central nervous system.

Establishment of awareness of function of the pubococcygeus is essential. No clinical results from physiologic therapy can be expected without activation of this muscle.

Resistive Exercises

Very few women who initially lack awareness of function of the pubococcygeus will be able to continue correct contractions of this muscle at home after instruction in the office. Since they are unable to coordinate their muscles through the usual reflexes, it is necessary to establish a connection between contractions of the pubococcygeus and the sense of sight. Also, unless given an opportunity to repeat their efforts under visual control, thereby noting any progress they may make, patients are apt to become discouraged. A simple, direct, and reliable means to overcome these difficulties is the Perineometer. The last phase of office procedure is devoted to instructing the patient in the use of this apparatus.

In addition to visual control, this instrument provides a means of contracting the perivaginal muscles against resistance. Resistive exercises of this type have proved most effective in all branches of muscle therapy for the correction of disuse atrophy and for restoration of normal function. Resistive exercises are designed to strengthen the pubococcygeus in all its components, especially the minute end-fibers which, in genital relaxation, have undergone atrophy. This muscle is not accessible to any other therapeutic measure, and its function is rarely improved by surgical procedures.

With the vaginal chamber of the Perineometer in place, the physician watches the manometer while the patient repeats for several minutes those efforts of which had been found to result in contractions of the pubococcygeus muscle. If the patient who had previously lacked normal awareness of function uses the pubococcygeus, only irregular and weak contractions can be expected. The indicator will show only a slight rise, between 1 and 5 mm. Hg.

The patient herself watches the manometer while continuing the same efforts. If contracting correctly, she is instructed to continue the same exercises at home for 20 minutes three times daily. In addition to these exercises, the patient is advised to repeat the same contractions without the apparatus many times a day. The more frequently correct contractions are repeated, the sooner will the muscular function be established as a reflex that does not require any further voluntary effort.

About 50 percent of all patients who start their exercises correctly will, during the first few weeks, lapse back into the old habit of using extraneous muscles instead of the pubococcygeus. Therefore, it is necessary to re-examine and re-instruct at weekly intervals for one month, and thereafter as often as necessary to insure correct use of the Perineometer. In this respect, a progress chart kept by the patients is of great value.

Complaints of fatigue, aching muscles of the back and abdomen, and nervous irritability following exercises are usually due to unnecessary use of extraneous muscles.

Objective Evidence of Improvement

In patients who exercise correctly and diligently, the following progressive changes will occur:

Establishment of awareness of function of the pubococcygeus.

Slight, gradual increase in initial manometric readings from a level of 1 to5mm. Hg. to as high as 20 to 40 mm.Hg. or more.

Muscular contractions can be felt in areas where none could be demonstrated before, especially in the anterior and lateral quadrants of the vaginal wall.

Contractions of the pubococcygeus which at first were weak and irregular became strong and sustained.

Improvement in tone and texture of all musculofascial tissues of the pelvic floor and outlet takes place.

Increased bulk of the pubococcygeus and its visceral extensions becomes evident.

Changes occur in the position of the perineum, introitus, urethra, bladder, neck, and uterus in relation to an ideal line drawn between the os pubis and coccyx.

The vaginal canal becomes tighter and longer.

The vaginal walls, which formerly were flaccid, improve in tone and firmness.

Bulging of the anterior vaginal wall (often diagnosed as moderate cystocele) becomes less pronounced.

Prolapsus of a freely movable uterus, when present, with cervix presenting near the level of the introitus is usually improved, and in some instances the cervix has ascended to as high as 5 to 7 cm. above the introitus.

Supportive pessaries, worn for as long as ten or more years, can usually be discarded without return of discomfort.

Patients can be fitted with smaller contraceptive diaphragms, whereas diaphragms of larger size formerly slipped out of place.

Therapy

Urinary Stress Incontinence

Muscle education and resistive exercise with the Perineometer produce dramatic results in the treatment of true urinary stress incontinence. This type of incontinence must be distinguished from urge incontinence caused by various pathologic conditions involving the upper urinary tract, such as infections, strictures of the ureter, stones, diverticula, developmental anomalies, etc.; incontinence due to fistulae; and spastic incontinence due to spinal cord changes following injuries, poliomyelitis, multiple sclerosis, etc.

In simple urinary stress incontinence, control of the urinary outlet is partially lost with coughing, sneezing, laughing, or other sudden strains. In the past, women tolerated this annoying and embarrassing condition with all its undesirable psychological effects because it was felt that the conditions did not warrant surgical intervention.

With physiologic therapy, complete relief from simple urinary stress incontinence has been consistently obtained in a series of over 700 cases of this type.

As some degree of awareness of function is initially present, the response to muscle education is prompt. Symptoms usually show improvement within two weeks after starting resistive exercises using the Perineometer. Lasting relief, however, depends on firm establishment of muscle reflexes and strengthening of muscular structures.

In severe urinary stress incontinence, dribbling is constant or intermittent. Patients with this degree of incontinence have ceased to make an effort to control the flow of urine, depending on pads and tampons. The normal reflexes of urination have been practically lost.

In these cases, because the pubococcygeus has been little used for many years, the muscle is atrophied. Often there is a history of so-called "bladder weakness" dating from childhood, aggravated by childbirth, severe illness, injury, menopause, senile changes, or pelvic surgery. Cases of this type have in the past been treated by surgical intervention, often with disappointing results.

The first step of physiologic therapy, muscle education, must be carried out meticulously and with great patience in this group. It is often necessary to repeat instructions at weekly intervals for many months.

Since these patients are trying to contract muscles which they probably have never before in their lives used voluntarily, they are likely to employ those of the abdominal and gluteal regions. It is therefore necessary to re-instruct patients carefully during weekly office visits and, at the same time, prevent them from becoming discouraged in their efforts.

As awareness of function and strength of the atrophied visceral end-fibers of the pubococcygeus returns, Perineometer readings will increase slightly and gradually.

Approximately two months of diligent exercise is required before improvement of symptoms is noted. In a few cases satisfactory relief was not attained until after a year of concentrated effort.

Severe urinary stress incontinence has been treated by physiologic therapy in a series of 212 patients, the majority of whom had previously undergone one or more unsuccessful surgical interventions to relieve incontinence. Good urinary control was established in 84 percent of this group.

These patients were able to discontinue the use of pads and have remained continent under normal circumstances. Recurrences have occurred after debilitating illnesses, prolonged spells of coughing, etc., but these could usually be controlled by resumption of resistive exercises for a few weeks.

While all cases of simple urinary stress incontinence were relieved, only partial relief or failure occurred in 16 percent of patients with severe urinary stress incontinence. These failures could be traced to local or general complications. Local conditions included marked shortening and scaring of the anterior vaginal wall due to previous surgical procedures or radium therapy. In three instances, however, good results were obtained following surgical release of restricting fibrous bands. Also, it appears that exercises of the pubococcygeus cannot succeed where the connections between this muscle and bladder neck and proximal urethra have been severed. Among the general conditions accounting for failures are neurologic changes, mental deficiency, senility and advanced diabetes.

When urinary stress incontinence coincides with a large cystocele, the incontinence is first relieved by active exercises and the cystocele corrected later through surgical repair.

Additional Measures in the Treatment of Urinary Stress Incontinence: Patients suffering from urinary incontinence usually have formed the habit of restricting fluid intake. In order to increase use of the bladder outlet, they are advised to drink at least 8 to 10 glasses of water a day and to interrupt the flow of urine several times while voiding. If successful, the contractions which resulted in interrupting the stream should be remembered and immediately duplicated during exercises with the Perineometer. The use of vaginal tampons and pessaries which exert pressure upon the bladder neck to control the urine is discontinued, since they interfere with the urinary reflex and contribute to atrophy of the pubococcygeus. For the same reason perineal pads to absorb the urine are reduced in size and eliminated as quickly as possible.

Genital Relaxation

The widest field of application of Perineometer exercises is in the treatment of genital relaxation during the childbearing and early menopausal years. While the results obtained are less dramatic than in the treatment of urinary stress incontinence, many more women (over 30 percent) complain of this annoying condition.

In the past, no conservative treatment has been available. Women in their child-bearing and most active years, therefore, had to endure discomforts and pelvic fatigue due to genital relaxation, usually described by the patient as bearing down, fullness, or "falling-out" sensations, until surgical intervention became advisable after the menopause.

This type of genital relaxation is recognized clinically by marked roominess of the middle third of the vagina and the presence of some degree of cysto-urethrocele, uterine prolapse, rectocele, and bulging or lax perineum. It has been found that these conditions are associated with poor function of the pubococcygeus, and that when function of this muscle is restored, complaints are often relieved and the clinical findings ameliorated.

Functional and structural improvement of the pubococcygeus has been demonstrated to have indirect influence on the support of the uterus. It has been observed that with increasing tone of the pubococcygeus the smooth muscle diaphragm, which is the chief support of the uterus, becomes strengthened - again demonstrating the pivotal importance of the pubococcygeus muscle.

Subjectively, patients describe relief of their complaints as feeling stronger in the pelvic, groin, and lower back regions and report that they are able to be on their feet for long periods of time and do their housework without having to lie down at frequent intervals.

Since the discomforts of genital relaxation are not as incapacitating as those in urinary stress incontinence, women in this category are apt to be haphazard in their exercises. It is, therefore, common experience that it takes longer before definite and enduring results are obtained. Diligent patients usually begin to notice symptomatic relief after 2 to 4 weeks of resistive exercises. Structural changes are, at this time, too slight to be palpable. In order to be of lasting benefit, exercises must be continued until improvement in tone and strength of the muscle can be clinically demonstrated.

Prophylactic Use

After the beneficial effect of resistive exercises on atrophy of the pubococcygeus muscle had been satisfactorily established, it was logical to prescribe Perineometer exercises before major degrees of pelvic relaxation had occurred.

Obstetrics

The usefulness of these exercises during pregnancy has been extensively investigated by Bushnell. His experience, which now includes more than 500 patients, indicates that about 30 percent of all pregnant women have a weak, thin perineum and poor contractions of the pubococcygeus.

By exercises with and without the Perineometer, the muscles become stronger, thicker, and firmer. Postpartum repair is facilitated, and fewer sutures are required. As soon as the effect of anesthesia has worn off, these patients are able to perform strong contractions of the perivaginal muscles, especially at the level of the middle third of the vagina. Pain and edema are less frequently observed.

The incidence of early postpartrum relaxation of genital muscles was greatly reduced. One would expect that in later years urinary stress incontinence, cystocele, urethrocele, uterine prolapse, and malposition of the uterus will develop less frequently in these patients. However, no definite statement to this effect can be made until after additional years of observation.

Taken as a group, young expectant mothers are most diligent in their exercises of the pubococcygeus muscle. Their cooperation is easily obtained once they understand the relationship of a strong pelvic musculature to sexual appreciation and the avoidance of later so-called female complaints.

Postoperative

The value of postoperative exercises for restoration of normal function has been firmly established in all other plastic and orthopedic procedures for repair of neuromusculofascial-tendinous structures.

Physiologic therapy of the pubococcygeus permits application of the same principle to surgical reconstruction of the tissues of the pelvic outlet.

Because of the great friability of the muscles, the surgery of the pelvic repair is limited to anatomic approximation of the fasciae. Whatever reconstruction of the muscles can possibly be achieved is incidental to repair of the fasciae.

Restitution of muscular function, essential to maintenance of the surgical result, can only be obtained by the subsidiary technique of active exercises of the pubococcygeus. Thus, these exercises are indicated following perineorrhaphy and in anterior repair to improve elastic support of the bladder, including all types of surgical procedures for the correction of urinary stress incontinence. As Collins has pointed out: "It is a good idea in all cases that have been operated on for prolapse of the vagina vault or uterus, or in every postpartal woman to teach them how to contract the vaginal musculature and let them use this as a prophylactic measure."

Conclusion

Experience with muscle education and resistive exercises of the pubococcygeus has proved gratifying whenever these procedures have been applied to conditions due to, or connected with, impaired function of the pelvic musculature. On the basis of therapeutic results achieved, it seems possible that other ill-defined complaints referable to the genital tract in women might profitably be studied from the standpoint of muscular dysfunction. For instance, it has been found that dysfunction of the pubococcygeus exists in many women complaining of lack of vaginal feeling during coitus and that in these cases sexual appreciation can be increased by restoring function of the pubococcygeus. The field of physiologic therapy of the pelvic muscles is thus much wider than at first suspected.

In the present paper, only the essential points of diagnosis and therapy of genital muscle relaxation have been presented.

References

Anson, Barry J. Atlas of Human Anotomy. Philadelphia: W.B. Saunders Company, 1950

Bushnell, Lowell F.: Physiologic Prevention of Postpartal Relaxation of Genital Muscles. West. J. Surg., Obst &

Gynec. 98: 66-67, February, 1950

Counsellor, Virgil S.: Methods and Technics for Surgical Correction of Stress Incontinence, J.A.M.A.46: 27-30, May 3, 1951.

Curtis, Arthur HJ., Anson, Barry J., and McVay, Chester B.: The Anatomy of the Pelvic and Urogenital Diaphragms in Relation to Urethrocele and Cystocele. Surg., Gynec. & Obst. 68: 161-166, February, 1939

Jones, Edward Gomer: The Role of Active Exercise in Pelvic Muscle Physiology. West. J. Surg., Obst. & Gynec. 58: 1-10, January, 1990

Kegel, Arnold H.: The Nonsurgical Treatment of Genital Relaxation, West, Med & Surg. 31: 213-216, May, 1948

Kegel, Arnold H.: Progressive Resistance Exercise to the Functional Restoration of the Perineal Muscles. Am. J. Obst. & Gynec. 56: 238-248, August, 1948.

Kegel, Arnold H.: The Physiologic Treatment of Poor Tone and Function of the Genital Muscles and of Urinary Stress Incontinence. West, J. Surg., Obst. & Gynec. 57: 527-535, November, 1949

Kegel, Arnold H.: Active Exercise of the Pubococcygeus Muscle. Meigs, J.V., and Sturgis, S .H., editors: Progress in Gynecology, vol. II, New York: Grune & Stratton, 1930, pp. 778-792

Kegel, Arnold H.: Physiologic Therapy for Urinary Stress Incontinence. To be published in J.A.M.A.

Kegel, Arnold H., and Powell, Tracy O.: The Physiologic Treatment of Urinary Stress Incontinence. J. Urol 63: 808-813, May, 1990

Read, Charles D.: The Treatment of Stress Incontinence of Urine. Meigs. J.V., and Sturgis, S.H., editors: Progress in Gynecology, vol II, New York: Grune & Stratton, 1950, 690-697

Collins, Conrad G.: Chicago Med., Soc. Bull. 241-246, October 13, 1931

About the author

Barry Fowler has had a lifelong interest in health, medicine and the environment even if his early career did not follow an obvious path in this direction.

In the decade after graduation from Queen Mary University of London with Honours in Physiology he undertook postgraduate studies in Economics, Business Management and Marketing whilst pursuing a business career that took him to the highest levels of in marketing management in several business sectors.

In the late 90s he met the inspirational entrepreneur Susie Hewson (see foreword) at a time when he was fundamentally reviewing his ambitions and lifestyle. He was very impressed with how she was trying to make a difference to the environment and to the health of millions of women and soon became heavily involved in a major campaign to promote the use of her biodegradable feminine hygiene products. He set up a new company to bring healthier and more environmentally sound products to a wider audience and began to import and distribute a wide range of cloth and natural hygiene products.

It was around this time that he began to write more extensively on health, fitness and environmental issues. His early research sparked an interest in the treatment of incontinence and began to raise questions about the way in which incontinence is managed both by the sufferers and the medical community.

So began a ten year campaign to raise awareness of the use of exercise to treat incontinence and some of the other common health problems that arise from childbirth and the menopause.

This book is the latest element of that campaign.

When not managing his various business interests Barry tries to pursue a healthy lifestyle. He can be found at the gym most days and practises Iyengar yoga regularly. He spends as much time as possible outdoors - skiing, cycling, hiking and camping according to the season.